The Ninjja Sutra

The Ninjja Sutra

Surviving the Health-Care Web

Neelam Phadke

ISBN: 1511446927
ISBN 13: 9781511446921
Library of Congress Control Number: 2015904828
CreateSpace Independent Publishing Platform
North Charleston, South Carolina

Contents

Introduction

"*Sharir madhyam khalu dharm sadhanam.*" This Sanskrit proverb says that the **body is the foremost instrument for fulfilling all the duties in life.** I heard this from my father ever since I can remember. Unfortunately, I had never internalized it until recently.

That said, we all want to lead healthy, fulfilling lives. Every individual has a different interpretation of what this means and entails. For some, this might mean finding time in their busy schedules for taking health supplements, doing regular health checkups, or going to the gym; and for some, this might entail leading a regimented life replete with yoga and meditation. For some others this might mean constantly fulfilling their taste buds through "healthy portions" of sinfully delicious food and hoping that their strong genes will take care of the aftermath of such excesses. I have personally moved around on this spectrum at different stages in my life.

The saying above takes the relevance of a healthy body to a completely new level; the first thing that should be taken care of is one's body; everything else follows. I learned this the hard way. Even for the enlightened ones among us, our pursuit of health is bound to take us at the door steps of the "health-care machinery" at some point. However hard we try, this is unavoidable. I use the term "health-care machinery" or the "health-care system" to cover a broad range of intertwined characters like the doctors, nurses, hospitals, insurance companies, pharma companies, funding agencies, and policy makers and how they affect ordinary mortals like you and me. To a normal person this might feel like a gigantic "web".

This is the only machinery (possibly after Fedex) that people place their utmost trust in. Jokes apart, I have seen doctors be revered like God, nurses considered the epitome of care and affection, health insurance a passport to good health, and hospitals the ultimate place for finding the elixir of health.

Yet, **the savior sometimes becomes the "terminator."**

All of us have stories to tell, ranging from relatively simple ones like a medicine that caused a strange reaction, a needle prick that became sore, or a simple beauty surgery that did not go that well to heart-wrenching tales of medical errors.

Despite billions of man hours and trillions of dollars spent every year, this machinery seems still very far from the six sigma standards that other industries measure themselves against. Although, there is lack of reliable data on medical errors globally, a WHO report that references various studies provides directional inputs on the prevalence and magnitude of errors –"Estimates suggest that as many as one in 10 patients in developed countries is harmed while receiving hospital care; in developing countries the number may be significantly higher. At any given time, 1.4 million people worldwide suffer from infections acquired in hospitals". It is a well-accepted fact that medical science is not foolproof. Part of the problem is the product itself—the human body, which is by far the most complex system on this earth. And often, this complexity becomes the ground for justi-fication, in case of unsavory outcomes.

This explanation alone may not be enough for some of us. We are talking about the life and the strong emotions of the people involved. As I witnessed a hospital getting vandalized (due to a perceived breach of trust) from the ensuing traffic jam, I couldn't help wonder if we needed to oscillate between such extremes—reverence to vengeance.

Yes, there are many gaping holes. This machinery, which can make the difference between life and death, requires a concerted effort to address serious challenges. But, given the complexity, even with the best intentions of all the stakeholders, this will take time. To top it all, if we add the complication of providing health care to billions of poor who can't afford to pay, the problem reaches a new magnitude. In the meanwhile, should we just wait?

I don't think so.

Several actions are under our control. Many pitfalls can be avoid-ed by the patient and his or her family through better awareness. If you are caught in a malfunctioning vehicle, repairing it shouldn't be your first line of defense; escaping with minimum injuries should be. That is indeed the focus of this book.

I have explored the challenges and practical solutions from the perspective of a receiver of health care, Ninjja, who is the main protagonist in this narrative. I have woven my own personal experiences, along with those of my family and friends whom I have had an opportunity to observe closely, into the form of a coherent story.

Let me introduce you to the two primary characters in this story, Ninjja and her father. They represent two ends of the spectrum: one is extremely averse to seeking medical help, and the other has a blind faith in anyone wearing a white coat.

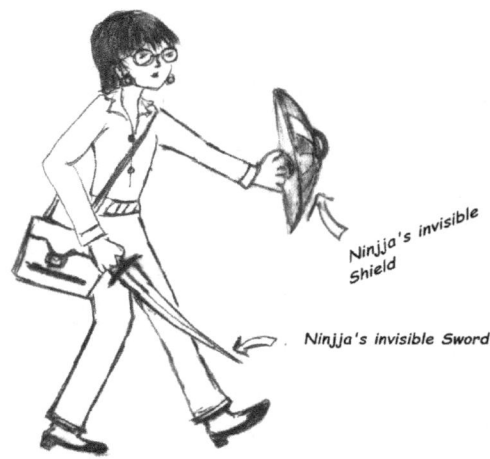

Ninjja: A working woman and a doting daughter. Has a fighting spirit and carries an invisible sword and a shield.

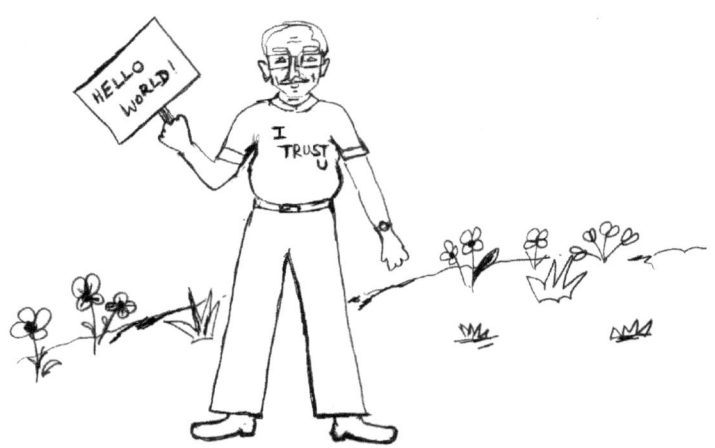

Baba: Ninjja's mild mannered father, who trusts everyone.

As destiny forces Ninjja to face the health-care system across two continents over a decade, she begins to see it as a drama played by comical characters but is surprised to learn how the behind-the-scenes crew plays an even bigger role than the more familiar cast. To keep the suspense intact, I refrain from introducing other characters in the beginning.

This story is an emotional roller coaster. Yet the point of view expressed is based on taking a dispassionate look at the situation and is complemented with research. For a management consultant, stepping back, keeping emotions aside, and analyzing issues objectively is a key requirement of the job. I have tried my best to use this training to disregard emotions and look at the issues objectively.

My goal here is to tell a story and share lessons, but often words fall short. To make this story come to life, I have made a pictorial representation of different characters who play a role in this drama. In my cartoons, I have dramatized the personalities to make the point. My intent is not to offend anyone from the medical fraternity.

For those interested in possible solutions for the health-care ecosystem, a starting list of actions that different stakeholders can take for betterment of this machinery is covered in the Appendix. I have tried to keep things simple, so that every single action can make a difference and doesn't need to wait for everything to come together at the same time. I hope that the sum of the parts will turn out to be bigger than the whole.

This book is meant for anyone who is either a receiver (a patient or a patient's caregiver) or a provider of health-care or someone who is in the pursuit of the enigma of health.

I hope that each chapter offers you some practical insights—either expose you to a new challenge of the health-care system or offer a practical tip to navigate the system to your benefit.

The pages from Ninjja's diary in the form of **My Survival Mantra** summarize the key lessons. At a later point, skimming through these eighteen pages can be an easy refresher.

Hopefully, you can go along with Ninjja on her journey and benefit from the bite-size pieces of practical advice she provides to survive the healthcare web. Let's start with "**the circuitous route.**"

One

The Circuitous Route

MARCH 2002

Ninjja was deeply submerged in her work when her phone startled her. It was her mother on the other end. She was trying very hard to sound calm and confident, but the timbre of her voice told Ninjja that something was not right.

"What's wrong? And please...please tell me the whole truth," Ninjja probed in a concerned tone.

"Well, there is nothing serious, and you should not worry. It's just that your dad is not feeling too well after his cataract operation." Her mother paused, possibly to gather some courage, and then continued. "He seems to be in some sort of trance...he is not in control of himself."

Her mother's convoluted explanation confused Ninjja even more.

"What do you mean, he is not in control? What is this trance? I don't understand!"

Then, Ninjja heard another voice. One of the friendly neighbors had decided to take charge and cut to the chase.

"Listen, Ninjja…your father is lying down with his eyes closed and speaking continuously and incoherently. It is impossible for anyone to understand! We can't even figure out what language it is…he is clearly not in his senses. He can't even get up or eat or drink on his own, but he won't stop talking. No matter what your mother says, I think you should come here."

This was too much information for Ninjja to absorb. She took a deep breath and asked the obvious question: "What does the doctor say?" The answer did not offer her any further enlightenment except for the consolation that her father was receiving medicine.

The whole situation was unlike any other incident that Ninjja had ever heard of. She felt like a kinetophobic person who had been pushed onto a giant wheel. She had a lump in her throat, and her head was spinning. Her father was suffering from some undiagnosed issue, thousands of kilometers away, and here she was…in the middle of a grueling project where taking out even fifteen minutes from the day was enough to make her team leader nervous.

She had to decide while still on the giant wheel! Fortunately, her heart made the call for her without wasting much time…she had to be with her father. Ninjja tried to take control of her anxiety and started figuring out the fastest possible way of getting to her parents, located in a small town in the state of Uttar Pradesh in Northern India.

After several hours of hectic activity to get the logistics under control, when Ninjja finally got on the plane, she couldn't stop wondering what had gone wrong in such a harmless, simple procedure as a cataract correction. Incessant blabbering? It did not make any sense. Why wasn't any medication working on him?

Having spent nearly five and a half hours for the two-hour flight (considering horrendous local traffic and flight delays), she was already feeling tired at the start of the next leg of her journey—a six-hour drive from the airport to her hometown. The manic taxi driver who aggressively meandered through the single-lane highway dotted with villages with no electricity didn't help Ninjja's already agitated nerves. She had to try very hard to keep her eyes off the road (or the lack of it!) and focus on the issue at hand—her father's condition.

Finally, when she got home, the sight of her father was more pitiful than what she had imagined. He was lying on a bed surrounded by over a dozen worried relatives and friends. Most of them were perplexed, while some were amused by his continuous blabbering. He had been in this state for the past forty-eight hours, and the physician's visits and medication weren't making any difference.

The family had to struggle to push even a couple of spoonfuls of soup through his mouth. Offering any solid food was impossible, as he had forgotten how to chew. *Forgetting to chew?* That was something Ninjja hadn't imagined even in her worst fears. When Ninjja tried to converse with her father, he recognized Ninjja's presence for a split second and then went back to his trance.

Needless to say, a couple of other doctors were also consulted, but they also gave a false sense of comfort by saying, "Give it some more time." Ninjja couldn't understand how everything could be left to "time" when no one even had a plausible explanation of what was going on.

Ninjja and her mother were at their wits' end when a brave family friend, who wasn't afraid of being chided for suggesting something that was considered a social stigma, came up to Ninjja's mother and said, "Shouldn't we be calling in a psychiatrist?"

This was a completely different angle that caught the family by surprise. Ninjja's mother exclaimed, "What? A psychiatrist? Why? I don't understand…"

Ninjja wasn't too far behind. "Oh! Really? My father has one of the sharpest brains that I have ever seen. Can he suddenly lose his mind? How? This is impossible."

"Well, assessing whether he can lose his mind shouldn't be your focus at this stage. Don't you know that the mind and body are interconnected? The fact that your father has no control over his body tells me that something could have gone wrong with the brain. Also, look at his speech…sounds like he is speaking in Sanskrit, but it is incessant and totally incomprehensible. Can't you see? There is no need to get embarrassed about this, Ninjja! What is the harm in consulting a psychiatrist also? Nothing else is working, in any case," their friend responded.

This explanation sounded reasonable. With no other clear options in sight, Ninjja and her mother decided to give it a try despite their apprehensions.

Within an hour or so, the psychiatrist was in their home, examining Ninjja's father. For once, Ninjja was thankful for being in a small town, both for the shorter distances as well as for the courtesy of the doctors. In a metropolis, several hours would have withered away before one could even get face-to-face with a doctor. The math was very simple: one hour for an ambulance to pick up the patient, one hour on the road, and another hour or so for the hospital procedures and waiting time before one would be graced with a doctor's presence. This arithmetic, of course, did not account for the ordeal of moving around with a patient who had no capacity to even move his head!

Ninjja was expectantly watching the new doctor. The psychiatrist took a good look at her father and appeared unperturbed. He took the incessant blabbering to be as normal as a physician would take a slightly raised pulse rate. He suggested that the first step was to calm the nerves of the patient. His hypothesis was that a wrong nerve had gotten pressed during the cataract procedure. The second possibility was that there was some other subclinical problem that had gotten triggered during the surgery. In either case, his first point of defense was to administer some pills to work on the nerves.

As expected, the medication wasted no time in putting the patient into a deep sleep. There was a sudden silence. Her father wasn't blabbering anymore!

The collection of neighbors frittered away in no time, as a sudden stop had been put to all the action. A few close family friends stayed back in the spirit of solidarity. Soon, seconds turned to minutes and then to hours. It was like watching a suspense movie where the slow motion of a few scenes really gets on the nerves. Ninjja was beginning to get worried by her father's immobility, when suddenly he opened his eyes.

He was awake, and yet he was quiet! Ninjja immediately jumped to his side and called out for her mother. It seemed like he was making a special effort to even move his eyes. His eyes finally caught Ninjja, and she could see a glint of excitement. He was definitely aware of his surroundings then. Gradually, he was able to recognize everyone and spoke an intelligible, normal sentence: "I am hungry...please get me something to eat." Everyone in that room gave a long sigh of relief. This new normal state felt like a dramatic transformation, given the starting point that everyone had witnessed.

Despite her father's inability to function without any support, the family embraced the change as a sign that the situation was redeemable.

The doctor was glad that he had found the right direction. The medication continued to work, though the root cause remained elusive.

Despite the tremendous drowsiness that came as baggage with psychiatric medicines, Ninjja could see that her father was on the path to recovery.

· · ·

After two days, Ninjja was back on the plane again, but her mind couldn't stop reliving the whole experience. Finally she took out her diary to give an outlet to her emotions. She jotted down her experience and then started wondering—How come a trusted regular doctor couldn't figure out that the patient's problem was not a physiological one but was in the realm of psychiatry? It was strange that one had to go with the hunch of a layperson instead. What could possibly explain this? Was he worried about the social stigma attached to visiting a psychiatrist and wasn't sure how the family would take it if he were to recommend this option? Or was he unaware of the limitations of his own expertise?

Soon, she was thinking about the trend of "specialization" in the area of medicine. Wasn't it possible that one could get too lost in one's area of focus? It could blind a doctor from seeing linkages with other parts of the body and mind. Possibly, the general physician was concerned only with the physical indicators and ignored the role of the brain in this whole mess.

The answer possibly lay somewhere in between these options. There was no way of knowing the truth without broaching an uncomfortable conversation with the doctor.

She kept tossing different thoughts in her head till she realized that knowing the truth really didn't matter. What was important was to be able to find one's path even when everything around was hazy.

What if she had asked the doctor a few follow-up questions? What if she had asked around to see if there were any other ideas? Why did she just shut her eyes and assume that the regular doctor knew best? If this concerned family friend hadn't made the suggestion of calling in a psychiatrist, Ninjja's family might have still been lost in the woods. She had learned her lesson. She took a fresh page and made a note of her key lesson.

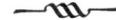

My Survival Mantra

1. **Don't assume that your regular doctor will always know what is right for you. Your two best friends should be exploring and asking! Believing in one's doctor is a good thing, but one needs to watch out for this belief turning into a blind faith. If the treatment doesn't seem to be moving in the right direction or something looks**

amiss, one needs to explore more. There is no better way of exploring than to ask relevant questions of the attending doctor. The next line of questioning should start with close friends and family. Exploration is not devoid of confusion-but it can enable one to see a different perspective to tackle the same issue and hopefully result in a better outcome!

—ɯ—

While Ninjja found a solution for the future that was within her control and was the best bet in the absence of a systemic solution, she continued to think of the underlying challenges that this particular episode had exposed her to.

A flight attendant announced that it was time for everyone to switch off their electronic equipment to prepare for landing, and Ninjja smiled to herself. For a change, she wasn't tied to her laptop; her thoughts didn't need any switching off, nor did they have to be reined in a seatbelt. She decided to use the last twenty minutes to jot down the challenges that this experience had brought to the fore and opened another fresh page in her diary.

—ɯ—

A receiver's perspective on health-care challenges

I. **Death of the quintessential family doctor:** Old Bollywood Hindi movies often showed a "doctor saheb"¹ who had a relationship with the whole family-someone who understood the psychological constitution of each person and not just the physical symptoms. This doctor was able to guide (and sometimes also chide) them through the medical maze as required. These days, either one finds "superspecialists" who have forgotten that other body parts also exist and interact with each other, or there are overzealous GPs (general physicians) who sometimes don't know where to draw the line and refer the patient to the expert. With a plethora of technological and scientific advances, is the fine art of judgment fading away?

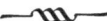

Ninjja paused to think about the experiences of her extended family and friends that she was aware of. Fortunately, with adequate digging, she could find some gems of excellent judgment that had saved significant physical and financial drain for many of the people she knew. *But where are such doctors now? How does one find them?* She was probably looking for a species that was becoming extinct. She scribbled the last sentence before returning her diary to the bag.

The plane had reached the parking bay, and it was time to find the taxi driver, get on the conference calls, and start the frenzy of work. Her work module was frozen in time from four days ago, and

---

1 *Saheb* is a term of respect (equivalent to "sir") used in India after the name. The origin of this word dates back to colonial India.

now it was time to play a mega catch-up game for the board meeting that was coming up early next week. Despite a stressful time on the personal front with almost negligible sleep over the last few days, she immersed herself into work with gusto as soon as she got to her desk. The day zipped past her. It was two in the morning, and she decided to follow the signal given by her body in the form of a headache to call it a day.

The following day, when she started again at seven in the morning to beat the traffic, the headache was still there. It was going to be another long day, and Ninjja decided to pop a pill to take her through the day. She needed to go on.

The meeting went off well: the analysis and presentation were appreciated, there was a lot of discussion, new questions got raised, and no decisions were made!

At last, it was time to get a good night's sleep and get ready for the next major meeting coming up in ten days. Fortunately, the long commuting time in the congested city offered enough opportunities for Ninjja to call her parents and check on her dad's health. She had been getting a consistent theme of good news on her father's recovery.

· · ·

APRIL 10, 2002

It had been over a month now, and Ninjja was hoping to get a declaration of full recovery sometime soon from her parents. But when she spoke to her father in the morning, she found his voice extremely feeble. He got tired after talking for just couple of minutes. This was enough to get her worried again.

Gradually, she learned that he had been struck by a fever with chills ten days back that waned after a dose of antibiotics. This information had been cleverly concealed from her to save her some anxiety. There were no signs of a fever, yet the weakness was increasing day by day. In the spirit of being doubly sure, one other well-known doctor was consulted too. However, even the new doctor couldn't find any signs of fever or any other ailment.

The consensus across the two doctors was that the weakness was the side effect of psychiatric medicines, and it would go away with time.

Ninjja was at a loss. The sudden increasing trend of weakness didn't seem to fit with this theory.

Why should the weakness increase with every passing day? Some side effects of the psychiatric medicines, like drowsiness, are well known, but is it possible that the medicines that are supposed to work on the brain start playing havoc with the whole body? Why didn't he feel such weakness in the first few weeks, when the psychiatric medicines were started? Something doesn't seem to fit!

She didn't dare ask for more time off from work to attend to this new complication. Above all, she wasn't sure if her time off would do anything to change the situation. Yet, something had to be done… but what?

Later that evening, when Ninjja was racking her brain on what to do about her father's health, Arv (her old friend) called. She needed someone to talk to, and the timing of this call couldn't have been better.

"Arv, what would you do in this situation?" she asked after an initial preamble.

"Well, I presume you don't believe that your little town has all the best doctors that this country has to offer...I would call them here and consult a good general physician for a second opinion," was his authoritative reply.

"That is impossible!" Ninjja exclaimed. "There is no way my dad can do a six-hour car ride and then catch a flight to get here."

Arv was not prepared to take no for an answer. "Who knows? Someone might have started a plane service in the last few weeks. The least you can do is to check it out first...if not, then we may have to think about other complicated ways of getting him here. Now, go and try." He signed off as though this were the last option available on this planet.

Ninjja thought about it some more. Despite sounding preposterous, the idea did feel worth a try.

As luck would have it, a flight from her tiny town in Uttar Pradesh to Delhi had just been started, and it was possible to take another connecting flight from there to Mumbai. The hopping round-trip was going to put a sizeable dent in her supposedly handsome monthly income, yet the information felt as soothing as the first shower of monsoon season. After some hesitation, she bought the tickets and sent them to her reluctant parents.

· · ·

Finally, after another week, when her parents arrived, her dad was in a wheelchair and was unable to even get into the car without help.

Ninjja hadn't expected the situation to be that bad. She was even more concerned now.

Given this condition, it didn't make sense for her to take them to her apartment, where they were going to be alone for at least twelve hours on any given day. Ninjja quickly decided to stop the cab in front of her aunt's house, which was a ten-minute detour from her own apartment.

As expected, her aunt was all too excited to receive her sister (Ninjja's mother). As soon as they had settled in, Ninjja's uncle declared a state of emergency and took the matter into his own hands.

"I don't think we need to wait anymore. I have a doctor friend next door who has a pathology lab. I am taking your father for a comprehensive blood test."

Given his authoritative style, Ninjja wasn't left with much room for argument. Above all, just a needle prick and some cash outflow as a downside didn't feel like reason enough to take on a bulldog. Everyone nodded in agreement.

The test results arrived the following day. Sure enough, the lab tests indicated that something was wrong. The commander in charge decided to hop across to another doctor in the vicinity. After a physical examination and a few additional lab tests, the diagnosis was given as "subclinical double malaria and typhoid." The word "subclinical" caught Ninjja's attention.

"No wonder the thermometer never gave away his condition!" she exclaimed as her uncle relayed the information nonchalantly. What surprised her the most was that none of the doctors back home had asked for these specific blood tests.

"Do the doctors of smaller towns rely on the physical indicators and their own judgment a lot more than they should? Or are they overcautious about their patients' ability to pay for the expensive laboratory tests? Or is it a question of limited exposure?" Ninjja found herself hurling innumerable theories into thin air.

Before Ninjja could go on any further with her internal debate, her uncle started to talk about the doctor's advice. The doctor wanted her father to be admitted to his small hospital to start the treatment immediately. Given that the problem had gone undiagnosed for several weeks and was leading to atrophy, the advice seemed reasonable. In a city like Mumbai, proximity to home was an important consideration. Instead of hunting for branded hospital chains, the family decided to go with this small hospital in their vicinity.

· · ·

After three days or so, one could see signs of recovery. Ninjja's father was definitely feeling better, and the blood tests were looking good, too. This small hospital had no meal services, but thanks to the courtesy of Ninjja's uncle and aunt, they got their regular home-cooked meals during this time. *Why does one need to even struggle for basics?* Ninjja wondered. What if she didn't have any relatives to support her? Managing meals while one was taking care of a sick patient was no joke! And not to forget, there was work, too, which consumed most of the day and the night.

Ninjja had to get back to her complex demand-supply model, so she put the brakes on her frustration and started focusing on her Excel sheet instead. When the 10:30 a.m. tea arrived, she was done with her analysis; now was the time to convert it to a presentation. After an hour or so, Ninjja found it very hard to concentrate; her sleepless nights in the hospital were getting to her. The effect of the tea had withered away, and Ninjja thought of getting some fresh air.

When she got back to the hospital later that night, she got the good news that her dad would be released after a day. She couldn't contain her big grin that night. Her father was also in an incredibly chatty mood, which lifted her spirits even further.

Finally, on day five, when the family was all excited at the thought of leaving the hospital, the doctor arrived with a new blood report and announced, "We will need to keep him for another week. We will be starting the treatment for TB (tuberculosis) from today. His condition is very fragile, and we can't take chances. We already have him on the drips and can easily use the intravenous drugs for better effectiveness." His manner was dictatorial and didn't leave any opening for even a single question.

Ninjja could see that even her mother couldn't believe what she had just heard. She was quick to point to Ninjja that her father was clearly looking better, and that the treatment for tuberculosis was lengthy. There was something that didn't feel right. While Ninjja was grappling with the nerve-racking thought of a continued stay in the hospital, she heard her mother's voice in the background "We need time to think about this; please let this treatment wait for another day."

Ninjja was glad that her mother had managed to buy some time for them to think.

In all this confusion, Ninjja got delayed for her client meeting by fifteen minutes. Her boss, Al, was livid, and Ninjja thought to herself, *That's it! This could be the end of my career in this firm!*

Unsurprisingly, the client didn't arrive until ten additional minutes later and offered no apology (it was easy to blame all the delays on traffic). If nothing else, it allowed the much-needed time for Al's temper to cool off.

Later that evening, as Ninjja was closing her laptop to head out to the hospital, she saw Al standing behind her desk. "I came to apologize," he said. "I didn't know that your father was in the hospital. Sorry about my outburst this morning...let me know if we can do anything to help you." Ninjja found his gesture very reassuring.

She told herself, *Ninjja, dear, looks like you still have your runway. It does seem like the top rung still has its soul intact, unlike in the* Dilbert *comics, where the moment one becomes a manager, the devil takes one's soul.*

Later that night, her family was divided on starting the TB treatment. Ninjja's uncle said, "So far, this doctor has been good, and we have seen improvement under his treatment, so let's just follow his advice. There is no point in taking chances."

Ninjja's mother had a different view: "This treatment lasts several months and can't be stopped in between. What if he doesn't have TB? The medicines will make him weaker and may hurt him more."

Finally, given the severity of the new treatment, they decided to seek one more opinion.

The next day, despite serious protests from the doctor, who refused to even sign the release form, the family stood by their decision. Ninjja communicated their intent nicely but firmly: "Doctor, please try to understand. I think my father will do better if he could be at home. We would really like if he could take rest at home for couple of days before starting round two of hospitalization. We take full responsibility for this decision. Can we please take him home now?" Finally, the doctor had to give in.

Now it was again Ninjja's job to talk to her friends and colleagues to find a trustworthy general physician. It wasn't easy to reach a conclusion, as there were many confusing caveats attached. Ninjja wondered if there was a way to organize all this information sitting in people's heads for easier access. "There are only so many people one can talk to for forming a conclusion within few hours. Clearly there is a lot more rich information available out there, if only one had the time, energy, and resources to tap into it!" she muttered while going about her search for "Dr. Right."

Finally, through some inexplicable equation, she zeroed in on one doctor and managed to secure an appointment for the following day.

Ninjja's parents undertook the arduous one-and-a-half-hour journey through the dust, smoke, and honks of the crazy traffic to meet this new doctor. Luckily, Ninjja had a shorter ordeal to deal with, as her office was closer to the doctor's clinic.

As Ninjja looked at her father, she wasn't sure what had caused him more exhaustion—uncertainty about a presumed illness or the never-ending mad traffic.

After a long wait, they were finally ushered into the doctor's office.

Ninjja had already organized the case file and studied the reports, and she was ready with her quick summary for the doctor even before he had started his examination. The doctor listened to her intently for the next five minutes and then asked, "Are you also a doctor?" as though giving testimony to her capability to synthesize.

"Well…I am a management consultant," she blurted. The doctor looked as surprised as she had been at his comment a few seconds ago. She felt compelled to explain, as the doctor still had a quizzical look. "Simply put, I wade through qualitative and quantitative information to find insights and synthesize them so that decisions can be made. I guess what I do for a living came in handy today." The stiff-upper-lipped doctor smiled at her response.

Fortunately, he did not get alarmed by the one data point of ESR (a test that signals inflammation due to infection in the body) that had led the earlier doctor to hurriedly get into the mode of starting treatment for TB. He spent quality time in examining the patient and asked many probing questions.

Ninjja was already feeling good even before the doctor had given any conclusion. The doctor finally gave his view: "I don't see any other symptoms. High ESR can also be a temporary phenomenon because of old age. Let's watch the trend over some time before we start any treatment. For all you know, it might just go away naturally."

Such a response was a great consolation. Ninjja kept her fingers crossed for the final "all-clear" signal, which was still a few months away.

After two weeks, the laboratory results of the ESR test showed a declining trend, and a follow-up test after a month confirmed the same. There were no other accompanying symptoms like cough or fever. Ninjja shared an update with the doctor, who was equally glad to see that his judgment call had proved right.

"You must be relieved. Your father doesn't have TB. Just ask him to eat well and sleep well," said the doctor, who seemed to have formed a good bond with Ninjja.

With steady improvement in her father's health, Ninjja's parents felt that they were ready to go back home. Needless to say, within few months, the ESR became normal without any medication (and, more importantly, without any hospitalization).

. . .

Ninjja was on her way back after seeing her parents off at the airport. The events over the past eight weeks did a quick replay in her head. She hit the "pause" button at one event: the "TB episode."

What was the hurry to start a new treatment? Clearly the doctor would have known that the treatment was lengthy and that unwanted medication would do more harm than good. Was it just an error in judgment, or had greed gotten the better of him? Why couldn't he wait for a reconfirmation of the diagnosis through further observation? Why was he so reluctant to release her father from the hospital? A plethora of questions started boggling her mind. To ease her confusion, Ninjja tried to put herself in the shoes of the doctor who was running the small hospital, and scribbled down the pros and cons of this decision from the doctor's perspective.

Pros and Cons of a new line of treatment from the doctor's perspective

Pros	Cons
• Additional immediate revenue from the hospital stay (at least Rs. 25,000, or US$500) • Follow-up consultation charges • Revenue share from follow-up tests • The consequences of the wrong treatment wouldn't be severe enough to kill the patient.	• Long-term damage to health of patient through unnecessary medication (some of it might not be visible in the short run) • Financial loss for the patient • Inconvenience for the patient

Probably the error in judgment had happened in weighing the pros and cons. The weight attached to the pros helped the doctor cross the line of the patient's trust and the ethics attached with his profession. Probably the violation of ethics all around had affected his behavior as well. *Should we be holding doctors to higher standards of ethical propriety when every local and international newspaper is replete with stories of corruption and its deep roots in India?* Ninjja wondered. *Is the pain and damage caused by building a faulty bridge any less than that caused by damaging a patient's health through unnecessary hospitalization or medication? Then, why should we be shocked if a doctor breaches our trust?* One difference, though, was that whenever incidents happened with bridges, it grabbed the headlines, whereas most health-care-related incidents went unnoticed.

There were no easy answers to these questions. Ninjja's mind inadvertently did a quick scan of her experiences with different professionals and service providers—contractors, builders, plumbers, electricians, teachers, civil servants, government bodies, doctors, and hospitals, to name a few. What was the level of honesty one found across all those categories?

In her sample, she saw a silver lining: possibly, the percentage of individuals who were able to uphold their intellectual and moral integrity was still in the double digits in the medical profession, compared to the decimal points in several others. She was terrified to think of the day when the medical profession would also stoop down to the benchmarks set by some others.

Ninjja continued her mental comparison of the medical profession with others and tried to stretch the corollary for her own curiosity. *For other professions, structured methods have come up to factor in the costs of "loss of integrity" in financial terms—i.e. through inflated budgets. The second-order effects of occasional loss of life and destruction of national wealth find only sporadic mention and are rapidly erased from people's memories. Aren't we stretching the envelope of being known as a tolerant society to an extreme of apathy and depravity?* The more she thought about it, the more disgusted she became. *To incorporate a similar trend in health- care, should we be making systematic provisions (similar to the financial ones) for loss of health and life and moving on? Is it OK to assume that some people will pay with their lives for the few others to fill their coffers, or is it high time we* woke up? *Is the soul of the health-care machinery being governed by dark forces?* Ninjja's vivid imagination created a dark figure that she named "SOULMAC". She saw this dark form as the soul and the primary driver of the health-care machinery. Soaked in greed and invisible to normal humans, it lurked in the background to maximize profits at any cost.

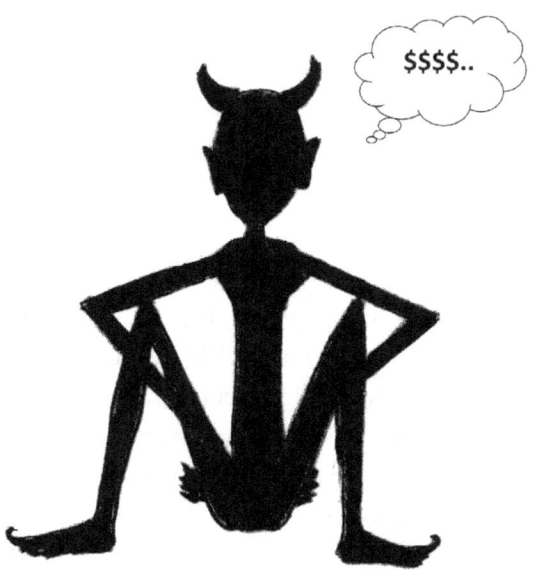

**SOULMAC: He is the soul and the primary
driver of the health-care machinery**

•   •   •

The taxi stopped in front of her building, and as she dived into the bottomless abyss called a "ladies' bag" to get cash, out came her yellow diary instead of the wallet. It was a signal to pen down her thoughts. She couldn't wait to get inside her apartment and was already scribbling when the elevator stopped.

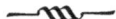

A receiver's perspective on health-care challenges

1. Death of the quintessential family doctor

2. **Moral corruption spreading its wings in the medical profession?** It is very naïve

to assume that all the health-care providers will always act in the best interests of patients and will never give in to the temptation of maximizing immediate gains. Revenue targets from the hospitals or personal priorities may drive a doctor to make a dubious interpretation of what is right for the patient. Our lack of awareness can make us even more trusting. Unfortunately, one may not even realize that one has been cheated or robbed. It is hard to isolate the challenge from the general moral fabric of society, but are we willing to compromise on the sanctity of certain relationships, such as that of parent and child? Where does the doctor-patient relationship sit in our hierarchy? Fortunately, the good apples still outnumber the bad ones, but the outcome of running into a bad one in the health-care world could be life-threatening. There is no reliable way to find out if one is being taken for a ride. Given the rate at which incidents of violation of patients' trust are increasing, this is not a challenge to be shrugged off!

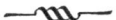

Ninjja didn't have perfect solutions to address the above concerns. She had some sketchy ideas—but she was sure that she hadn't unearthed all the challenges, and neither did she fully understand all the root causes.

Trying to solve a problem that wasn't even fully defined was not something she thought even a genius should attempt. However, she firmly believed that one could certainly control one's own actions. She chose to fall back on this belief to establish a starting point. *Is there something I can change in my actions as a receiver of health care till the perfect model emerges?* Her reflection shed some light on the ways and means to mitigate risks to some extent. She started scribbling her thoughts again.

My Survival Mantra

1. Don't assume that your regular doctor will always know what is right for you.

2. **When in doubt, seek a second opinion, especially in situations where the new treatment is going to be tedious or long or can have serious side effects.**

   The key question then becomes, how does one identify the second source in the absence of any structured information? People may give their opinions based on their experiences, which may or may not be relevant in one's situation. Select probing questions can help understand the rationale behind the views and help in forming one's own judgment regarding whom to consult for a second opinion:

   1) Why do you think he or she is a good doctor? (This helps in understanding if the recommendation is being made

on hearsay or based on personal experience.)

2) What was the issue you were facing when you consulted this doctor? (This helps in assessing the similarity and complexity of the situation.)

3) How much time did the doctor spend in reviewing your situation and understanding the context? Did he or she ask questions related to your general health? (This helps in determining if the doctor takes a comprehensive approach and assessing his or her interest level in the patient versus in maximizing the number of patients seen per hour.)

4) Did this doctor suggest anything different? Did he or she explain the rationale? (This indicates that the doctor is confident enough to form his or her own opinion in a logical way.)

5) Which other experiences do you have with the same doctor? (This is to get a sense of repeatability.)

6) Was the doctor approachable during the course of treatment? (This helps assess the ease of course correction should there be any side effects or complications.)

7) Which institution is the doctor attached to? (Attachment to a reputed

hospital signals certain minimum standards. This is good to have, but it is
in no way sufficient in the absence
of 1-6 above.)

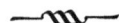

Two

Money Matters

MAY 2002

Ninjja was feeling energized after a final review presentation with the client. The chairman listened with rapt attention, and one could see that he was getting clarity around options for future direction. The meeting ended with an indication of a follow-up project.

During the minicelebration that followed, the senior partner showered his benevolence upon the team and offered the next day off. Probably the magnitude of his largesse would have been different had he known that over the past three months, the team had been working till three or four in the morning with no weekend breaks.

As Ninjja hit the sack that night, she could feel that every bone and muscle in her body was aching. The adrenaline rush from the great meeting had ended. Her willpower had lost its grip over her body, and now it was reeling in deep protest. "I guess I have been stretched a bit too much due to Dad's illness, along with this harrowing project. I will be fine tomorrow," Ninjja told herself as she closed her eyes.

When she woke up, she had a high fever. She had had her share of visits to the doctors and the hospitals over the past three months and was in no mood to see a doctor unless someone convinced her that she was going to die. Sleeping and eating became her best friends over the next two days, and somehow they managed to drive away the fever.

When she reached her office, she was surprised to find that other members of her team were also sick. *What a coincidence!* Ninjja thought. *Did we all catch the same bug at the same time? Or could this be due to the stress?* The latter idea was so repugnant that she quickly brushed it aside. *Why should there be any stress when one has enjoyed the challenge?* That was what everyone was told during the orientation program. *Something that signals weakness can't be a probable cause. Idea dropped! Case closed*, she told herself, and she started working on the proposal for the next phase.

• • •

OCTOBER 2002

Thanks to the client who didn't want to pay for the full team and the eagerness of her firm to accept this engagement as God's gift during the global downturn, Ninjja had an opportunity to enjoy a bigger challenge—being the lone warrior on the project! Although she would have loved to have some company, this wasn't bad, either, as the client team actually had the pressure to deliver. She quickly adjusted her orientation from being the doer to someone who gets the work done from an underequipped team. Ninjja was learning the art of breaking a complex problem into bite-size pieces that her team could chew on. Above all, she was discovering that without having a renewable source of patience, she was not going to survive the next six months.

The pain and pleasure of any work is equally a function of one's mind-set as it is of the content itself. Ninjja was doing just fine in this innovatively structured project.

While she was finishing her review that evening, she got the good news that her cousin had been blessed with a baby boy. This was a reason enough to lift her spirits for a hearty dinner.

. . .

The celebratory tone had just been set when her cousin learned that the newborn was sick.

The baby was still in the hospital, and the young mother was robbed of the moment that she was so looking forward to—holding and cuddling her baby. She had bottled up all her emotions and was praying for the dark days to be over soon.

With every passing day, they were swinging between hope and despair. The neonatal ward held the key to their little treasure.

Five days later, when Ninjja called her cousin, he sounded very despondent. Ninjja didn't know how to lessen his pain. For want of anything better, she hid behind a plethora of comforting words, as is the last resort of a person unable to provide any meaningful help to change the outcome.

. . .

Soon, the life support system had to be called upon. Ninjja's cousin and his wife pulled in all their resources to put up a brave fight and continued to pay for the exorbitant costs of the ventilator and the dialysis. Alas! There were no signs of progress.

When he asked the attending doctor on his prognosis, his response was, "This is in God's hands. Who knows, the baby may come out of it just fine."

The unspoken question that the young couple was facing was, how long would the waiting game continue?

After putting in twenty days and more than 5 lakhs (~US$10,000), the call was taken to withdraw the life-support system and end the suffering for the baby and for everyone around.

The tragedy finally ended, but it had left a deep emotional and financial hole.

Ninjja could certainly feel the handiwork of "SOULMAC"—the dark soul of health-care machinery—in aggravating the misery.

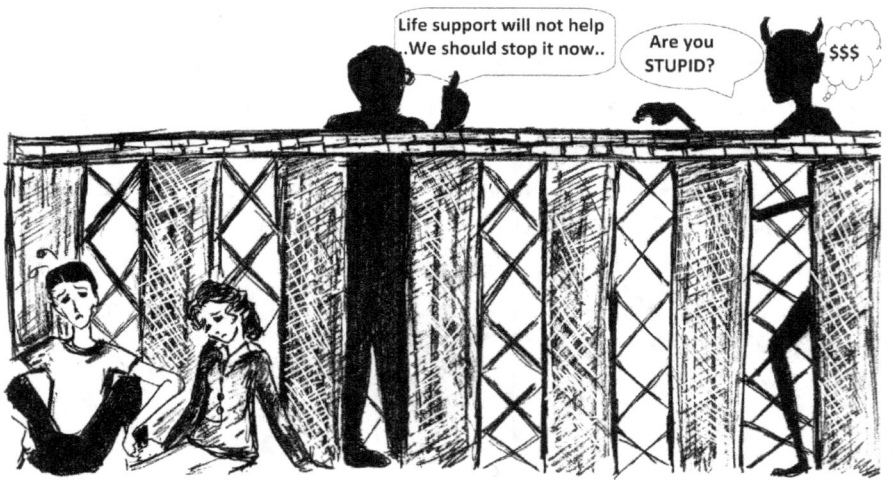

Terminally sick infant in ICU

· · ·

JANUARY 2003

Time is a great healer. Ninjja's cousin had come to terms with his loss, but the financial hardship was hitting him hard. The amount he had borrowed from the market to fund his hospital expenses was still

looming over his head. His monthly cash flow from his fledgling business was not adequate to fund the high interest charges he had to pay.

When Ninjja heard about this issue from her parents, her immediate reaction was, "Didn't he have health insurance?"

Back came the reply from her mother: "Who has? We've never
had it all our lives."

"Well, that's a good point. I used to think you didn't have an
insurance plan because you were above sixty. There are some talks,
though, that this age limit might move to seventy."

"Yes, it's too late now," responded Ninjja's mother remorsefully, wondering why no one had ever educated them about the value of health insurance. She cut short her reminiscence and said, "The good news is that
our extended family has decided to pool our money to salvage the debt
situation that your cousin is in. You can make your contribution as well."

Ninjja was happy with the family's decision and thanked God
for giving them the resources and the will to help each other. What
would happen if a truly destitute person ended up in this situation?
She learned from her friend that the penetration of health insurance
was below 10 percent in India. In more developed countries, this
number was in the range of 60 to 90 percent. The penetration in other emerging countries like China and Brazil was somewhere between
25 and 60 percent. Given that out-of-pocket expenses accounted
for over 80 percent of health-care costs, it seemed very easy for a
health-care crisis to push a household to bankruptcy. In addition to
the issue of affordability, lack of awareness as well as ease of usage
seemed to be the key roadblocks in India. "Even for people who
take the insurance, how cashless is this cashless support?" Ninjja
asked her friend who worked in the insurance industry.

"In practical terms, a large chunk still needs to be shelled out up front, and then one has to wait for it to be reimbursed later," her friend explained.

"What if the person can't cough up the dough up front?" Ninjja was perplexed and continued to feel overwhelmed by the shocking statistics that her friend kept throwing at her.

This seemed to be a sizeable enough challenge to merit a separate page in Ninjja's yellow diary.

—m—

A receiver's perspective on health-care challenges

1. Death of the quintessential family doctor
2. Moral corruption spreading its wings in the medical profession
3. **Affordability of health care**: The challenge of affordability becomes starker in the context of poor countries. The World Bank reckons that in India, which is not the poorest country in the world, 68 percent of the population lives below US$2 per day. How do we expect such people to pay US$50 to US$200 per day in hospital costs in their hour of need? Couple this with the poor penetration of medical insurance and the unavailability of smooth cashless transactions, and a large section may have to go without treatment or suffer at the hands of unscrupulous moneylenders. No

wonder health-care costs are believed to be the number-one reason for bankruptcy of rural people in India. As if the disease or the accident is not problem enough, there is a more lethal concoction waiting for the victim on the road to recovery.

—◆—

The doorbell interrupted her musings. Ninjja's aunt and cousin (who lived a few blocks away) were there to seek her help.

"Do you know anyone at the insurance company X [a very reputed name]?" Ninjja's aunt asked in a melancholy tone.

"Well, yes—why?" Ninjja responded quizzically.

"They are refusing the reimbursement of our hospitalization expenses, and we have fought enough…I am really tired now. Can you help?" her aunt asked helplessly.

Wow, what timing! Ninjja said to herself. *Looks like the issues go beyond just awareness and affordability. Someone who has bought insurance is not secure enough!*

Without wasting any additional time on thinking about the complexity of the issue at hand, she reassured her aunt that she would do her best to help her.

Now it was time to get to the execution. It wasn't as easy as she had imagined it to be. Ninjja had to use her network, in addition to a great amount of persistence and her training in arguing skills.

. . .

Finally, when the issue got as close to being sorted as it could be, Ninjja's aunt was relieved to get the partial payment. This process of getting the claim was also a process of discovery for her. She learned that there was fine print that covered the insurance company. The print could be read only with a magnifying glass, and no one had bothered to explain this to Ninjja's aunt during the selling process.

Ninjja had just gotten introduced to one more character in the health-care saga that she had started to unravel. Ninjja labeled this character the "Insulator"—the cool insurance company that has an inbuilt insulation against grievances. It is trained to kick away any claims that make an attempt to come its way.

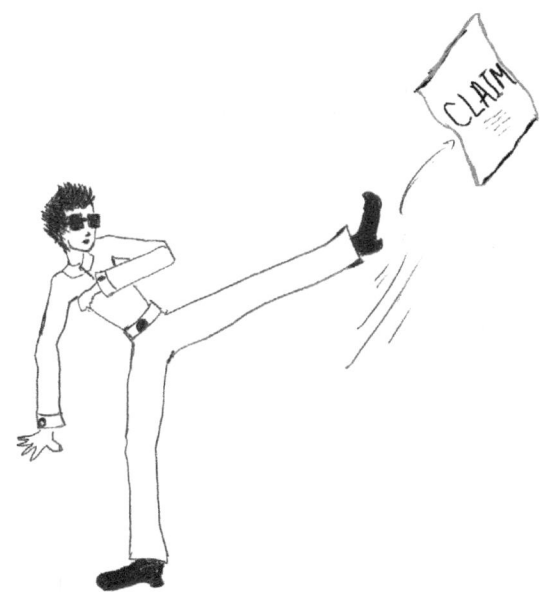

Insulator: The cool insurance company. Has in-built insulation against any grievances.

Later that night, Ninjja couldn't come to terms with the goings-on of the past few weeks with the insurance company as a normal course that one should get used to.

Her mind was racing, trying to put some logic behind it.

"Whether one should call this misselling or blame it on the naïveté of the customer can be a matter of debate. However, the fact that there was a gross expectation mismatch combined with mistrust for health insurance in general was a reason enough to sit up and take notice," Ninjja wrote in her diary.

Ninjja's aunt came out much wiser after this experience but vowed not to renew her policy. She wasn't even sure whether buying insurance from another firm would be worth the effort and money anymore. What was the economic value of this transaction?

Benefits	Losses
• Insurance company got revenue, which otherwise it may have lost (had the customer been aware of the fine print)	• Higher transaction cost for the company—more time and effort for claim processing meant lower profit margins on this transaction • No future revenue from the customer and no referrals • High stress (leading to long-term health issues) for all the parties involved

The answer to this equation—that there was no winner in this game—seemed very obvious to Ninjja but probably not to several others who seemed obsessed with doing just one transaction. *Are the white collars any different from cabbies who choose a longer route or tamper with the meter to increase the bill without giving a damn about their reputations or the value of repeat business? Possibly for a cabbie, it is always about one single transaction, but can any enterprise keep running with such a mind-set?*

Ninjja's cousin's experience of financial distress due to a medical emergency told her that her aunt's model of shunning insurance was also not the way to go.

It wasn't preposterous for Ninjja to think that a systemic solution was needed. Given the volumes of thought papers on this subject, she hoped that the future would sort itself out. However, she couldn't disentangle herself from the subject without penning down some suggestions for lesser mortals like herself who had to exist in the current times.

— ∞ —

My Survival Mantra

1. Don't assume that your regular doctor will always know what is right for you.
2. When in doubt, seek a second opinion.
3. **Always have health insurance and carefully select the plan:** In developed countries, obtaining health insurance is a no-brainer. In India, although everyone is mandated by law to insure his or her vehicle, no such stipulation exists for health insurance. Even the aware consider health insurance as an option, not a necessity. As in the developed world, make sure that you and your family have a health insurance at all times–either

through your employer or self-purchased. Given the ambiguous selling process, you must be very careful in selecting the plan and know what you are signing up for. Ask enough questions while taking your policy, and read it thoroughly, including the smaller fonts. Often, there are conditions that may prevent you from claiming the benefit when you need it the most (e.g., inability to claim any benefit till minimum tenure is complete, exclusion of certain ailments, exempting preexisting conditions, failing to renew within time-limit sets the clock back, and so on). Speaking to competing policy providers is a good way of figuring out what one lacks with respect to the other. You are then better informed to exercise your judgment. If you are pushing sixty and don't have a policy yet-it's time to act now! At a later age, when you may need the most health-care support, you may not find any provider willing to talk to you.

—w—

. . .

NOVEMBER 2002, MONDAY, 8:15 A.M.

Ninjja was excited to get back to the office after a long weekend and was looking forward to catching up with her friends. Unfortunately, at that hour she found only the pantry boy and the cleaning staff for company. With no other option in sight, she ordered her daily dose of tea and chocolate cream biscuits and settled down at her desk.

Around 9:15 a.m., her colleagues started trickling in. Remains of the Monday-morning blues after a long weekend could still be seen on their faces. Ninjja came out in the hallway to greet her friends. "So, did you all have a great time?" This trigger was enough to get everyone started. There were so many stories that were just waiting to be shared. Words started flowing as though a glacier was suddenly exposed to the Delhi heat in the month of May.

By the time she got back to her desk, an e-mail was awaiting her. She had to start a new outstation project the following day.

• • •

FEBRUARY 2003

Ninjja was thoroughly enjoying herself on the new project. Taking 15 percent out of costs wasn't easy, but the committed team and a driven CEO were making it happen. The day's hard work was well rewarded at the sumptuous buffet spread almost on a daily basis at the five-star rated hotel where they were staying.

Life was going well except for some minor irritants that Ninjja experienced—occasional headaches and minor knee pain while climbing up the stairs. All these indicators she summarily ignored while the project continued at a brisk pace.

• • •

APRIL 2003

Ninjja was getting ready for a review meeting at the client's headquarters, but her trousers wouldn't let her in. She had ignored the signals given by her belt buckles, and now she was literally stuck. Her backup formal dress that was supposedly loose and that she had termed as a wrong buy came to her rescue—it managed to just accommodate her. The traffic situation was fortunately on her side this time, and despite the mini fiasco, she still managed to reach the meeting in time.

"Ninjja, we need to rush up; the meeting starts in five minutes," her teammate, Rohan, exclaimed as they were climbing the stairs to get to the meeting room.

"I am trying hard, but my knee hurts," Ninjja shouted back in pain. During the tea break, Rohan picked up the issue of her knee pain and advised her in his usual grim tone, "Don't take this lightly. This could be arthritis or osteoporosis, and you can get into serious trouble."

"Are you mad? This doesn't happen at my age," Ninjja retorted.

Rohan had his logic tree fully worked out. He sealed the argument with a confident statement: "I know someone who is suffering from this at the age of twenty-six…so, the age really doesn't matter! You should not ignore this. Please consult an orthopedic ASAP."

The rest of the meeting was a washout for Ninjja. She had nightmares of herself walking with a stick and then moving around in a wheelchair. She knew that there was no way to reverse the onset of these diseases. After the meeting, she frantically called her friends to find a good reference for an orthopedic. Ninjja's mind had already started drawing vivid pictures of multitudes of tests that she would need to undertake, the frustrating time that she would need to spend running around the hospitals, and the innumerable lifetime medicines that she would have to consume. Needless to say, she wasn't too pleased with what she saw. In this moment of dejection, she was suddenly struck with a new idea. She remembered the doctor (a general physician) whom she had gone to for a second opinion in her dad's case. The very next moment, she was making an appointment with him for Saturday.

. . .

On the scheduled day, Ninjja felt the nervousness that she used to feel on the day of exam results in school. Feeling like the student who knew that he or she wouldn't deliver according to their parents' expectations, she managed to squeeze into a corner of the fully packed waiting area. Ninjja discovered that the appointment was only for that day and not a specific time. The pleasant secretary was totally inept at providing any sense of what Ninjja's position was in the waiting line or how long it would take. Fortunately, an adequate supply of film and glamour magazines helped in keeping her mind off the issue of her knee. She was fully up to date on all the Bollywood gossip when she was finally summoned in after one and a half hours.

. . .

Once she was in the office, contrary to the latest trend, the doctor spent quality time in understanding the history and nature of the pain. Ninjja was glad to see that the doctor was still as consistent in his approach as he had been a year ago when she had met him with her father.

To Ninjja's surprise, the doctor didn't stop at just understanding the nature of her pain. He tried to understand the lifestyle that Ninjja led (including travel, etc.) to put everything in context. Then he proceeded to get Ninjja to do a physical drill. Ninjja hadn't seen this coming, but she politely complied. It consisted of multiple rounds of sitting down on a very low stool and then getting up, standing on one leg, raising herself on her toes, and so on. He was asking questions and observing closely. Finally, he stunned Ninjja with a strange question: "Have you always weighed this much?"

Is he hinting that I am fat? she wondered. Despite the "unaccommodating trouser incident" that week, Ninjja still looked fit and qualified for the "normal" category of the BMI (Body Mass Index). Grudgingly, she responded, "No…I used to be very thin—actually underweight—until recently. I have put on ten kilograms in the past year and a half."

The doctor nodded and then moved on to explain. "Based on what you are describing, it looks like your legs have had to suddenly bear twenty percent more weight than they have ever done before. To top it off, your thigh muscles are weak…hence, your knees are feeling the pressure. Here is what you should do. I will teach you some exercises that you need to do religiously, and wear flat shoes as much as possible. Please wear a good knee support if you have to go for long walks, and don't forget that your posture during flights is very important. I suspect that your legs don't touch the floor when you are in the plane. Use your bag as leg support in the flights…and in the meantime, try to reduce your weight a bit. We will review again after six weeks."

That's it? No tests? No medicines? No regular visits to physiotherapists? Ninjja mumbled to herself.

• • •

Everyone else whom she narrated this to had the same reaction. Her well-wishers advised her to see the bone/knee specialist rather than take chances. Ninjja was witnessing the other side of the coin—a doctor who doesn't have tests and medicines in the prescription invites doubt. A large portion of advice was related to lifestyle management in this case.

Ninjja had developed a strong belief in this doctor and in his process of deduction. She had yet to see a doctor with such minute observation and questioning power. Also, the course of action that he had recommended made perfect sense to her. She decided to go with her belief rather than the popular wisdom.

. . .

Within a few weeks, she could feel some improvement, which encouraged her to keep going on the same path.

. . .

Ninjja was getting out from the cab for a follow-up session with her doctor when her phone rang. "I need your help urgently...I am in trouble," Arv squeaked from the other end.

"If you are not dying, can I call you in five minutes?" asked Ninjja, as she continued her financial transaction with the cab driver. After marking her attendance at the doctor's reception area, she proceeded to call Arv back and kill the ample time available till the rendezvous with her doctor. She had a hunch that this call was about matters of the heart.

After a long-winded prelude, Arv came to the point. "Well, there is this girl I like. She is smart, good-looking, good-natured...we have a great time together..."

So far it sounded familiar (except the "good-natured" part), and Ninjja had begun to wonder where the trouble was in this happy story.

Arv continued in a grave tone, "Now I think she has started getting serious about me."

Ninjja was perplexed. "Where is the problem? So far you were taking tips about wooing girls, and now you are worried! I don't get it."

"Learn to listen, Ninjja. I said 'getting serious'—that's where the trouble starts. I don't want to hurt her," Arv retorted.

"Brilliant. Why do you have to flirt if you are so afraid of commitment? Either back off now, or learn to get serious—don't think there is a third choice available to you," Ninjja responded, irritated.

"Why can't it be just the way it was? No steps backward or forward." Arv was not prepared to let it go. This was an interesting thought and made her pause.

The doctor was calling her, and she had to quickly make up something to close the call. "Because there is nothing static in nature…" She hung up with a promise to continue later.

•   •   •

JANUARY 2004

Ninjja had totally forgotten about the knee pain, but the exercises had become part of her routine. On the weight reduction front, there wasn't much progress to rave about. The weight was as immovable as some of her adamant corporate clients. However, she was proud that she had hit one major milestone as a proof of her recovered knees: she had managed the seven-kilometer dream run at the Mumbai marathon. Though she was among the last few to cross the magic line, the feeling of covering the distance more than made up for her abysmal performance on the dimension of time.

She called her mother in an excited state to inform her about her feat.

"You should be thankful to your doctor for giving you the right advice," was the first response from her mother, which sent her into a flashback to nine months ago.

• • •

This highly capable and reputed doctor had a fantastic revenue creation opportunity for the whole system—the medicine value chain, the test laboratories, the physiotherapists, and the like. There was an overly worried patient who had the ability to pay and would have been the perfect candidate to contribute to their coffers. Instead, he used all his experience to form the right judgment keeping patient's best interests in view and didn't bother about profit maximization. Ninjja was glad that she had gone with her instinct and trust rather than the label of a specialist.

She was glad to see living proof of the "knowledgeable, righteous doctors with excellent judgment," a species that was almost extinct. She just hoped and prayed that such a species, which she fondly christened as "Doxtinct," could be saved from extinction.

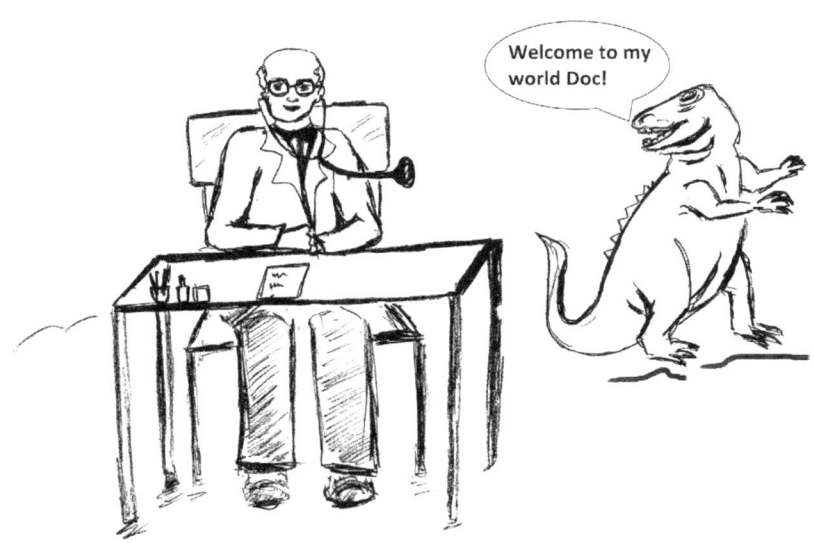

Doxtinct: He is knowledgeable, has patient's wellbeing as primary goal, and goes the extra mile. He is in grave danger of becoming EXTINCT!

Was there a new lesson for her in this experience? Was it in conflict with her first lesson? Ninjja thought about it and concluded, *Certainly, there is a new perspective that this experience has brought about. Whether one switches over to the specialist from a GP or consults a GP in a seemingly "special problem" is entirely dependent on the context. There is no reason this lesson can't coexist with my first doctrine. It is important to have an awareness of the situation so that the appropriate path can be chosen.*

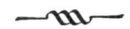

My Survival Mantra

1.   Don't assume that your regular physician will always know what is right for you
2.   When in doubt, seek a second opinion.

3. Always have health insurance and carefully select the plan.

4. **Don't rush to a specialist based on your perceived issue.** A good general physician whom you trust can be a good first point of contact. Try to understand the connections of the symptoms that you are facing and explore the root cause together. Use your judgment to see if the line of reasoning makes sense to you, and make your call. If the situation is not life-threatening, give it some time. Some diseases require changes in lifestyle and a sustained effort to see the results. Decide the appropriate time frame to review results along with your doctor. However, if the progress is not as per your expectation, don't forget doctrines one and two!

—⚡—

• • •

As Ninjja was opening the lock of her apartment, her phone rang. Tina, her first-ever roommate, was on the line. Unfortunately, she was no longer the chirpy Tina that she had known. Over the last couple of years, her calls had become less frequent and less exuberant. Tina's career as a banker was moving well; yet often, Ninjja could feel a melancholy undertone. She had an inkling but was afraid to probe about her married life. That day Tina opened up: "Ninjja, I still have nostalgic memories of our time together. It is ironic that I had a lot more sharing and fun time together with you than in my marriage. I don't know if this is due to highly demanding jobs, crazy commutes...or is it my inability to be the model daughter-in-law?"

She paused for breath and then continued, "My parents think that I have the perfect, happy marriage. Knowing the truth will break their hearts. My in-laws know that things are not going well and want me to have a baby as a 'solution' for sorting my marriage. Can you believe it?...The weight of pretending to be happily married is breaking my shoulders. How hard should I be on myself to keep everyone else happy?" Her voice trailed off.

Ninjja was mostly the silent listener in this conversation, but even after they hung up, she was so moved by Tina's plight that she couldn't stop thinking.

I am sure Tina is not the only one who has this burden. How about several other men and women who are carrying this weight due to the pressure to conform to societal norms and don't even have any other outlets, like a good career? That crushing weight must be creating stress somewhere in the system—that's the basic law of physics!

Is that the reason women are expected to have infinite resilience (the equivalent of elasticity in physics) and are trained since their childhood to save them from breakage?

It's surprising that we don't report the highest number of cases of depression and heart attacks—my guess is that these go unreported, she thought wryly. *Can the same Indian ethos, values, and close-knit families that keep people grounded become a source of stress? Do we ever think about the flip side of such an overbearing* attitude that totally ignores the issue of personal freedom? Why do we want everyone to fit the same mold?

There needs to be a line, and it is for every individual to define the limit for the breaking point. I really hope that Tina can soon decide where the line is for her, Ninjja said to herself as she opened the refrigerator to find something that could pass as dinner.

. . .

"Listen, there is something that you should know. Mother has been suffering from migraine-like headaches for the past two days, and the doctor has suggested a MRI," Ninjja's sister informed her in an unperturbed tone. Ninjja had not been expecting such an event to remind her that her parents were in the United States with her sister.

Ninjja thanked her stars that she had prevailed over her mother regarding the overseas medical insurance despite the grand discourse on her ironclad health.

A day of panic followed.

. . .

The highly anticipated phone call came in the morning, and the same cool voice informed her, "There is no reason to worry; she just needs to take some BP [blood pressure] medicines."

"How much did the MRI and doctor's fees cost?" Ninjja asked out of curiosity.

"Fourteen hundred dollars," was the matter-of-fact reply.

Though there was a sense of relief that her mother was fine, the price tag was enough to throw Ninjja off her chair.

. . .

Three months later, Ninjja received her beaming parents at the airport. After a few minutes of sharing their experiences in the great United States of America, the topic quickly moved to the heavy-duty MRI expenses. "I feel bad that your sister had to foot this bill," her mother started off.

Anticipating the direction such a conversation might take, Ninjja quickly cut it short by saying, "You don't need to worry. This will be reimbursed by the insurance company." Thanks to the immaculate file organization done by her brother-in-law, Ninjja didn't have to sweat over filing the insurance claim. All the paperwork was in order, and the claim was peacefully submitted.

A month went by, and there was no sign of the much-awaited check. Now Ninjja's mother was getting very nervous, and a daily call pushing Ninjja to follow up had become the order of the day.

Ninjja tried her best to pass on the irritation she felt during the morning call to her insurance providers, but they seemed heavily insulated. After several high-pitched shouting matches, the file started moving, and finally she heard from the insurance company: "This was a preexisting condition, so we won't be able to reimburse this claim."

Though there was no reason to believe that the headaches were a preexisting condition, Ninjja knew that now she had to prepare herself for the semifinals of the shouting matches.

Finally, the reluctant insurer offered to call up the family physician to confirm the presence of this preexisting "fictitious" disease. In a world of the disappearing breed of family physicians and innumerable patients that a doctor sees in a day, it would be a stretch to think that a doctor would recall the name, let alone the history, of a patient over the phone. There was no other option but to take this chance.

Ninjja thought about the concept of "prewiring"(getting an individual buy-in before the main meeting) prevalent in the corporate world and felt it wouldn't hurt to try it with the doctor in current situation. When Ninjja's mother called the doctor to give him a heads-up about the situation, he fortunately remembered that she had no history of headaches. This preliminary call certainly did its bit in preparing him better for the tricky call that was yet to come from the insurance agency.

As Ninjja learned later, the insurance call started with a preconditioning question: "Since when is Mrs. ____ suffering from headaches?" which possibly was a reflection of training and goals being set for them. The doctor was kind enough to handle the questions well, and his confidence removed all the barriers between the claim and the approval.

As Ninjja was about to find out, the finale was yet to come.

The system was showing the check as delivered, but Ninjja's family hadn't seen even a glimpse of it! Their detective work with the courier company revealed a fictitious signature of the receiver. How could she have forgotten about the pests on the way?

Fortunately, the insurance folks redeemed themselves by issuing a stop payment and handing over the new check in person.

Finally, eight months later, Ninjja's sister could reunite with the dollars she had spent for her mother's emergency tests.

Ninjja was curious about the statistics of the percentage of claims reimbursed in overseas medical claims. Irrespective of the numbers, her own experience suggested that the probability might be even less than that of a regular person climbing K2, the second highest mountain in the world that is thought by many climbers to be the ultimate climb.

Ninjja was struck with two major questions after this episode:

- What if you don't have a regular physician or have a non-descript personality that a doctor can't remember over the phone?
- What if the ailment is really serious, and you have to run up a huge bill? Borrowing to fund the treatment in the interim wouldn't be too farfetched. The long time for reimbursement and a good possibility of the claim being rejected can create serious havoc in the lives of people who are taking you in as guests. Are we supposed to take these policies just for mental peace and pray that we never need to call this option? Wouldn't we be better off just praying?

This seemed in sync with the insurance challenge that Ninjja's aunt had encountered earlier in the case of domestic treatment. The ethos of finding ways to reject the claim remained the same, but the potential of damage in the case of overseas insurance could be devastating. "At a minimum, people should be aware of this false sense of security that they hide behind while traveling abroad," Ninjja muttered as she picked up her pen.

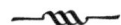

My Survival Mantra

1. Don't assume that your regular physician will always know what is right for you.
2. When in doubt, seek a second opinion.
3. Always have health insurance and carefully select the plan.
4. Don't rush to a specialist based on your perceived issue.

5. **Overseas insurance is not a blank check** to take care of your health-care needs when you are abroad. Use it for mental peace when you are in good health and if your hosts abroad are reasonably well-off. In other words, if you suffer from any serious ailment, think very hard before you board that plane. You might be exposing yourself (and possibly your hosts abroad) to a huge financial risk!

—⁓—

. . .

OCTOBER 2004

Ninjja wrapped up her work quickly to have lunch with her old friend, Amit, who was in town. After the regular buffet that one finds at all the good restaurants, Ninjja opened her purse and pulled out a huge pouch. Amit was staring at the pouch, quite bewildered. "Why the hell are you popping these medicines?" he asked.

"Well, I have to…eating out continuously causes major acidity, and I will end up throwing up if I don't have these pills."

Amit was at his sarcastic best. "This is interesting. You spend a bomb to eat out at the best places and then pop pills to digest the most oily and unhealthy picks that you can make from the buffet."

"What do you mean, unhealthy? I have to maximize the value from the buffet, so I pick the most delicious preparations to suit my palate," Ninjja retorted.

Now it was Amit's turn to fire all his ammunition. He was clearly way ahead on the learning curve of lifestyle and health. He quickly went through the "health quotient" of the fried snacks that Ninjja had savored and of the rich gravies and the multitude of desserts that she had gobbled in no time.

Ninjja's feeble protest of "But I don't take butter with my naan" didn't cut any ice. "Believe me, Ninjja," Amit continued, "as there isn't such a thing as returns without any risks, superdelicious food without any health risks is impossible. Compound this with eating out at odd hours every day, and you have a really lethal concoction."

"OK, let's concede that your theory has some merit, but how do you expect me to eat healthy when I am home barely one day a week?"

Amit was unstoppable. "Ha, I knew you would come up with such an excuse. Why don't you go back and have a look at the buffet spread, and tell me if you find things that would pass the lens I just gave you?" To Ninjja's surprise, she now noticed sections that had been nonexistent for her before. Soups, salads, boiled chickpeas, sautéed vegetables, dal (cooked lentils)—the list certainly wasn't short. Embarrassed, she agreed that she would try to control her natural gravitation toward the rich food.

"And don't forget that eating an early dinner is important." Amit threw in his last shot, now that he had proved a point. Given how fit Amit looked despite a grueling schedule, Ninjja was forced to pay some attention to his pearls of wisdom.

Ninjja had to rush back to her meeting, and Amit had to catch a flight soon, so it was time to say good-bye. As Ninjja was walking toward her office, she was amused that the lunch that day had given her more food for thought than the expected gastronomic delight.

· · ·

During the second half of the day, she had a tight schedule with back-to-back review meetings. While she was inadvertently munching on the chips and biscuits that were available in abundance in the conference room, a flash from the lunch discussion suddenly struck her. Did she really need to devour all the munchies, or was this a way to temporarily escape from the inane discussion that had completely taken over the meeting?

She immediately pulled back her protracted hand from the plate and tried to find her voice. Though this wasn't her meeting, in the interest of twenty other people who were silently suffering, she decided to take charge and steer the conversation in the right direction.

The meeting finally ended at seven in the evening. After that, Ninjja had to review a document her team had left behind for her input. Finally, at ten fifteen, when room service brought in her dinner, Amit's words came back to haunt her: "It's important to have an early dinner." She was about to brush it aside, given her work schedule, when something stopped her. Was it really beyond her control? Couldn't she have come back to the hotel after the review meetings, taken dinner, and then reviewed the documents? No one was waiting to act on her input that very night, after all! The futility of self-created work pressure was gradually beginning to dawn upon her.

Can't I try to have a healthier lifestyle at least 80 percent of the time? Ninjja asked herself, and she took on the challenge. She tried to educate herself on the linkages of lifestyle with health and started making her own set of rules. *Amit may have a more aggressive approach, but let me start with something that I can work with.* She wrote down her five rules for self-administration:

1. While traveling, avoid going for buffet spreads, as it is hard to resist the temptation of "sinful" food. Instead, settle for ordering "simple food" in room service. (She discovered later that some of the hotels and restaurants were comfortable not doling out the rich curries and did honor requests for "low oil" and "low spice" levels.)
2. I will plan my day such that there is no in-person meeting after 6:30 p.m. I will try to eat dinner before 9:00 p.m., and if I get delayed, I will survive on soup.
3. I will avoid eating during flights (except for breakfast, which is usually difficult to spoil).
4. I will try to carry fruits and nuts to the office to kill those mid-day cravings.
5. I will try to start my day with a glass of water and take tea or coffee without sugar (to reserve some calories for that sweet tooth).

It is typically hard to remember even three things without mnemonics, and Ninjja had set herself against a stretch goal of five rules. She tore this page out of her diary and pinned it on the board in front of her desk. Other Post-Its with tasks were fighting for space on the board, but Ninjja had made her five-point agenda immobile.

. . .

Two months had gone by, and Ninjja's dependence on antacid pills had totally gone. She felt a renewed energy. As an additional consolation prize, for the first time, she noticed the weighing scale's needle moving toward the left.

Now that she had achieved some positive results, the draconian discipline of the past few months seemed as easy as eating. The five rules had become part of her lifestyle, and she was indeed surprised that her hand didn't automatically gravitate toward the cookies and chips anymore. This was a moment of enlightenment for her, and she wanted to record her moment of truth.

My Survival Mantra

1. Don't assume that your regular physician will always know what is right for you.
2. When in doubt, seek a second opinion.
3. Always have health insurance and carefully select the plan.
4. Don't rush to a specialist based on your perceived issue.
5. Overseas insurance is not a blank check.
6. **A balanced lifestyle holds the secret of many a cure**. The definition of that balance is an individual's choice. Following everything that is written in the health literature makes it so daunting that doing nothing becomes an acceptable option. Investing time to understand the best practices and figuring out your own mantra will produce such dividends that you will never regret

it. The key is to know what is practical in your context, know what can have an impact (tweak it if needed), and then have the dedication to follow it.

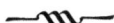

Three

Work, Mishaps, and More

JULY 2005

After her transfer as one of the first few employees to start a new office, she was getting used to living in new megalopolis—Delhi NCR (National Capital Region). Her old friend Raj, who thought of her like a little sister, made her feel at home and helped her settle in.

Ninjja was winding up her work when her phone rang. Arv's booming voice from the other end almost deafened her. "*You didn't even tell me that you have moved to my town!*" he screamed. After venting his frustration with her, he asked, "So, where do you live?" Ninjja felt a tad guilty for not informing her good friend about her move. To restore peace, Ninjja blurted out her address and said, "Let's meet up one of these days."

"Actually, I am in your area and can be there in forty-five minutes, if that works," came the answer.

"Fine," was the only reply Ninjja could manage before hitting the "sleep" button on her computer. She suddenly became aware of the fact that she had released her cab in the afternoon and had forgotten to make alternate arrangements.

To her surprise and dismay, everyone had broken the corporate code of working late every day and left before seven o'clock that day. After getting a "not available" response from all the local taxi providers, she was left with no option but to take the local transportation to reach home. It was going to be just a twenty-minute ride, so Ninjja happily made herself comfortable in a garishly decorated rickshaw.

However, she had grossly overestimated the road safety in her new city.

Her thoughts about taking this ride more often were violently interrupted by a strong pull on her purse. Two bikers managed to yank her purse from her, and the force was enough to land her on the concrete road with a thud. As Ninjja removed her hand from her throbbing head, she was horrified to find it covered in blood. The shocked rickshaw puller offered his headgear as a bandage, helped her back into the rickshaw, and resumed the journey. Ninjja was too stunned to tell him otherwise. A few moments later, she discovered that her cell phone was still in her hand, and she instinctively called Arv to check if he could come a bit earlier. Fortunately, he was just a few minutes away from her apartment building.

More surprises awaited Ninjja. After alighting from her ride for that evening, she found herself frozen on the ground. All her willpower couldn't help her move even by an inch. Completely exhausted with the ordeal, she resigned to the fact that she would need to be physically lifted to achieve any horizontal displacement. Arv was forced to test his weight-lifting prowess in the process of taking her to the hospital. In a state of panic, he took her to the nearest hospital that was mentioned by someone in the small crowd gathered to watch the spectacle.

Finally, eight stiches on her head and a few X-rays later, she was released with the advice to rest for three or four days. "You have been lucky. There is no fracture in your leg; it is just trauma from the fall. You should be able to walk slowly tomorrow," pronounced the doctor confidently. Ninjja was happy to see a minimalistic prescription with no "warning signals" or additional tests.

Two days had gone by, and Ninjja's claim to progress was that she could drag herself with the help of a cane for the bare essential chores. Arv offered to take her for a follow-up visit with the orthopedic specialist. The same message was reinforced with advice to "keep walking—a few steps at a time." Given her exceptionally slow rate of progress, Arv suggested that she spend some time with her friend Raj's family to recover and offered to drop her at his place.

• • •

Seven days later, Ninjja was back at work with a headscarf (to cover the bald patch that came as collateral damage along with the stitches) and a very visible limp. She had barely familiarized herself with the old environment when the next outstation project came calling. Traveling with an injured leg didn't sound sensible, yet Ninjja decided to take it on for fear of getting loaded with "pseudo work."

Ten days of literally dragging her feet around had taken its toll. While her mobility had increased marginally, the pain quotient had increased many times. Finally, she decided to fall back on her own doctrine of "second opinion" that she had been ignoring so far.

• • •

After doing some physical checks, the new orthopedic proclaimed that he suspected a fracture in the pelvic bone. The first X-ray drew in a dud (it showed no signs of fracture), but the doctor wasn't willing to let it go. A few explanations and iterations later, the technicians in the radiology lab got the angle right, and the doctor got what he suspected—multiple hairline fractures!

In an authoritative tone, he gave her two choices: "You can either get admitted to a hospital and be in a cast, or be at home but be absolutely horizontal for ninety-nine percent of the time if you don't want to limp all your life." Any normal human being would have taken the second option, and so did Ninjja. She promised to take time off for the next four weeks, secretly hoping that she might get well sooner.

Ninjja was thoroughly impressed with his skill as a doctor and chose to ignore his behavioral shortfalls. *I can certainly recommend him to my male friends*, she thought, and she hoped that she wouldn't need to go to him again for a checkup.

Although this new incident reemphasized her doctrine of "second opinion," she uncovered some of the popular myths as well. "If there is a fracture, it will show in the X-ray" totally ignores the fact that some fractures can be tricky to catch, and the doctor needs to be skillful enough to find it.

Finally, six weeks later, Ninjja was able to move about without pain, but the full recovery was still several months away. She was fortunate that the additional damage caused by dragging herself around (as per the first doctor's advice) wasn't irreversible. Being horizontal and staring at the ceiling had offered her ample opportunity to relive the episode after her accident. Was there a possibility of getting a correct *first* opinion? There could be many serious accident-related situations where a person might not have the luxury of limping around for weeks before going for a second opinion. How does one reduce the probability of damage?

Was there a fundamental issue with the quality of doctors in the emergency ward? She didn't have any other data points to tilt one way or the other. The sustained goof-up during her follow-up visit with the specialist was probably indicative of the quality of the hospital overall rather than any single individual. There was no magic wand that could be waved. The only thing that struck her was controlling panic. What if she hadn't been so dazed after the accident, and Arv hadn't gone into panic mode? Possibly they could have called a few friends to find out about good hospitals in the vicinity and driven a few extra kilometers to get to the right help. Hindsight is better than foresight, but Ninjja wasn't prepared to give up. *Even if some small tips could be stored and an even smaller percentage could be retrieved in the hour of need from our overloaded memories—it would be worth it!* Ninjja pulled out her diary to start scribbling again.

—w—

My Survival Mantra

1. Don't assume that your regular physician will always know what is right for you.
2. When in doubt, seek a second opinion.
3. Always have health insurance and carefully select the plan.
4. Don't rush to a specialist based on your perceived issue.

5. Overseas insurance is not a blank check.
6. A balanced lifestyle holds the secret of many a cure.
7. **In emergency situations (e.g., an accident), don't run to the closest hospital** that comes to your mind or gets mentioned randomly. In several situations, spending extra ten minutes to inquire about options available for medical help or driving few additional kilometers to get to a good hospital might prove worthwhile. Keep your regular physician's number handy-he or she might be able to guide you or make some calls to help you out. Additionally, ensuring that you have the contact details of some local person is a must if you are traveling. For those who have a "planner's mind-set," it may not hurt to have previous knowledge about good hospitals in the new area you are planning to visit or on your route if you are traveling long distances.

—⁓—

. . .

The forced time-out had also given Ninjja enough time to reflect on her own life as well as reconnect with her parents in a more relaxed manner. The self-imposed constraint of being indispensable for a project, which often forced her to push her physical limits, had come crumbling down. *The world won't stop if I die today, so why was I so hesitant to take even a day off when my body was screaming and begging for it?* she wondered. *Better late than never.* She vowed to listen to her internal signals with as much attention as she paid to the outside world.

Once at home, Ninjja started rediscovering other forgotten forms of keeping herself occupied, like reading books, getting her parents to fill in the blanks that she had about their lives, playing cards, and sometimes just doing nothing! In addition, she could credit herself with inventing the art of using a laptop while horizontal, the awkwardness of which provided plenty of entertainment to all the family and visitors.

· · ·

Ninjja inadvertently opened up a sensitive topic with her mother—her older sister. The death of her older sister had happened well before Ninjja was born, and she had heard only incoherent pieces of the event. She knew that the little girl was five years old…she had an accident at home…she was taken to the hospital…she would talk whenever she regained consciousness but didn't survive beyond two days…but Ninjja didn't know much about the exact sequence of events. Ninjja prodded her mother to fill in the blanks in the narrative.

After initial hesitation, Ninjja's mother got into the flow, and Ninjja was able to visualize and feel every moment of pain that her mother had felt thirty-five years ago. In some way, Ninjja was walking with her mother down memory lane.

Now, they were twelve hours into the hospital stay after the fateful incident, and Ninjja's mother was choking with emotions. "It was all my fault," she blurted.

Ninjja tried to calm her down with a gentle reminder that it was an accident. "You shouldn't blame yourself," she said.

Ninjja's mother was inconsolable. "No, I should have known; I should have been more careful. I had no idea what was happening." Now Ninjja had to push her to talk through the details of what exactly happened. Finally, she started talking again. "I was sitting by her bedside all night, waiting for her to wake up…she would blabber something and then go off to sleep…she was incoherent.

"In the morning I noticed that her bed was really wet, and I called in the nurse. The nurse came in and got into a panic—'Please don't say anything to the doctor,' she pleaded."

"This was even more nerve-racking. I later learned that the nurse hadn't connected the intravenous drips properly, and none of the medication actually went inside the body. To make it worse, air bubbles passed through the veins instead…it was a complete disaster! The doctor was called in frantically. He tried his best to salvage the situation for the next twenty-four hours…but the double whammy was too much for the little one to handle…and gradually she faded away."

Ninjja's mother stopped with a heavy heart, and the air suddenly felt very grim. Now the missing piece was falling into place.

Ninja could now see why her mother always avoided this topic. Her mother had been living under this guilt of not being able to spot the leak earlier in the night, but should she have? *Is a young mother with no experience of hospitalization expected to supervise a nurse?*

Ninjja's mind was still on the hospital scene, and she couldn't get over it. Maybe the injuries from the accident were so severe that her older sister wouldn't have survived, but didn't the little girl deserve proper treatment, at least? Didn't the nurse understand the implications of her callous behavior? After all, the "last mile" in any hospitalization depends on the nurses and attendants, and if they are underequipped, the consequences could be disastrous. A new challenge of the health-care system was staring at her now. She tried to overcome her emotions and turned to the scratch pad lying beside her bed to scribble a few lines.

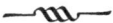

A receiver's perspective on health-care challenges

1. Death of the quintessential family doctor
2. Moral corruption spreading its wings in the medical profession
3. Affordability of health care
4. **Quality of attendants and nurses**: The final touch point that the patient has in a hospital stay is with the nurses and attendants. More often than not, the first line of contact or first line of defense is also with these important cornerstones of our health-care delivery mechanism. Efficient and correct delivery of treatment, along with immediate action in case of emergency, depends on these folks. But are they delivering on the responsibility they

are expected to shoulder? Reasons they aren't could be many-lack of training, performance monitoring, inadequate salary, and incentives, to name a few. An already haggard patient is the last person who should be expected to think about these issues and have a benign attitude toward callous slipups that can cost one's life! In a twenty-four-hour hospital stay, when a patient is seen by a doctor for less than an hour, isn't it high time to launch an effort to raise the quality of delivery for the other twenty-three hours?

Ninjja hoped that her mother's guilt pangs would be reduced to some extent by talking through it. However, that still didn't solve the fundamental problem that this episode raised—quality of the final caregiver. In her moment of frustration, she drew a caricature of the nurse, "NurSpOily," whose vivid visualization was refusing to leave her. This "NurSpOily" was capable of spoiling a good treatment and adept at the art of slipping away.

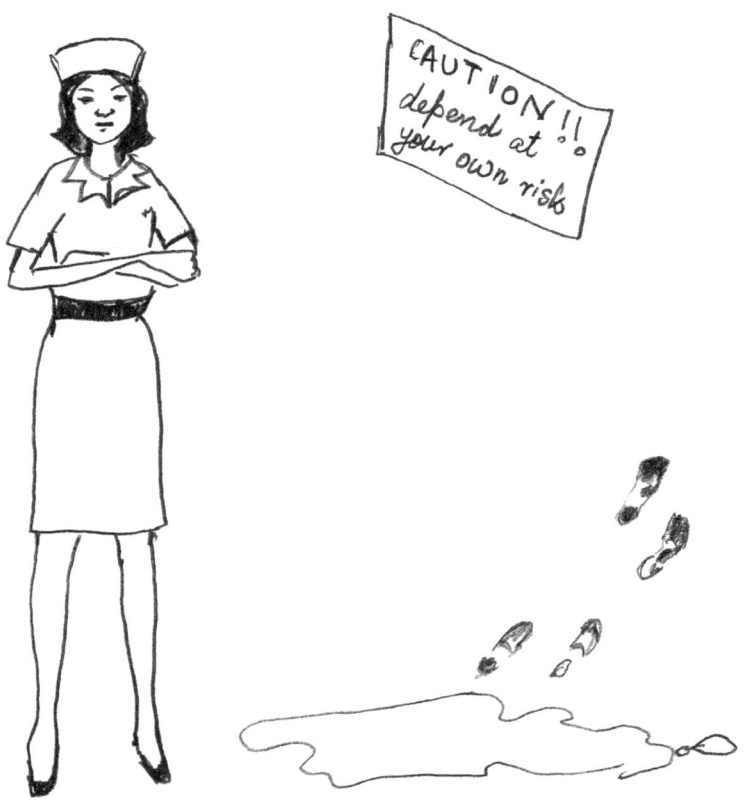

NurSpOily: She is tightlipped and finds it hard to move her hands from the comfort of being "cross-armed". She is capable of spoiling a good treatment. She is also "well-oiled" and is adept at the art of slipping away.

Ninjja continued to think about the underlying reason for poor quality of nursing staff. It was tempting to jump on the hypothesis of nurses being underpaid (compared to alternative opportunities for the same educational pool) and the lure of more attractive opportunities abroad as the key reason for the shortage of "quality nurses." Though this theory was not devoid of facts (e.g., the average salary for nurses was about a tenth of what their American counterparts would earn, which would need a stretch of imagination to justify even after throwing in the argument of purchasing-power

69

parity), there were several other industries that had managed to maintain service levels and quality standards despite similar salary differentials. Ninjja thought about the IT and BPO (business process outsourcing) industries, where the entry-level programmer or the data-entry operator earned much less than what the PPP (purchasing-power parity) comparisons would suggest, but the industry was able to manage the quality standards. Ninjja concluded that strong processes, project-management structure, quality audits and testing, training, strong HR practices, and strong adherence to service-level agreements (which were demanded by global customers) were the key differentiators. *Shouldn't we become demanding customers and create a pull for streamlining systems? Don't we check the expiry date of medicines before buying them? Then why should we settle for something that is below standard during the hospital stay?* Ninjja wondered. *However, this would work only if the information and feedback were transparent and if it materially affected the bottom line of the hospitals.* She signed off with this philosophical thought and vowed to think about something more tangible.

If nothing else, there was a lesson for everyone to be more watchful if their near and dear ones were to have a brush with the hospital bed.

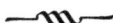

My Survival Mantra

1. Don't assume that your regular physician will always know what is right for you.
2. When in doubt, seek a second opinion.
3. Always have health insurance and carefully select the plan.
4. Don't rush to a specialist based on your perceived issue.

5. Overseas insurance is not a blank check.
6. A balanced lifestyle holds the secret of many a cure.
7. In emergency situations (e.g., an accident), don't run to the closest hospital.

8. **If someone dear to you is admitted to the hospital, don't assume that the nurses and attendants are always right.** Be vigilant regarding the injections and medications being administered. No one can stop you from checking them against the doctor's prescription. Ask about the different equipment that is installed, the meanings of different alarms, and whether there will be immediate action in case of alarms. Carefully monitor the sanitation standards, and raise an alarm if things are not up to the mark (several postsurgery and hospitalization complications occur due to poor sanitation standards or errors in administration of medication).

FEBRUARY 2006

Ninjja's career was moving well, and so were her responsibilities that came with her promotions. She hadn't found the mind space to think about the issues she had religiously scribbled in her little yellow diary, and she hadn't been able to find time for her passions in life. The only scarce resource in her life was time. The distinction between Sunday and Monday had blurred so much that sometimes she found herself habitually jumping into her formal corporate suit, which she jokingly referred to as her monkey suit, on a Sunday morning. One weekend she was working through the final board presentation when the doorbell rang.

It was half past noon, and it suddenly dawned on her that it was a Sunday, and Arv was coming over for lunch. She was visibly nervous as she opened the door to receive her visitor. As always, Arv was at his excited best and popped his head into the kitchen, saying, "I am starving…" He trailed off as he didn't see even a morsel of food or proof of attempting to cook anything.

Ninjja made a quick recovery with, "I was planning to order in," but Arv was smart enough to realize that she was making it up. He looked around, and the spread of papers and laptop on the dining table gave away the real state of affairs. He instinctively knew that Ninjja had forgotten about his visit. He tried to hide his disappointment with a fake smile, but putting up a facade was not his forte. The tension was apparent in the air, and they perfunctorily went through the chores of having their Sunday lunch. Ninjja was overwhelmed with guilt but couldn't muster the courage to apologize. She asked him to wait for evening tea, and out of politeness, Arv grudgingly agreed.

While leaving, he muttered, "Get a grip on your life, Ninjja." The comment bit her pretty hard and stayed with her all through the evening. Not being able to find time for the people she cared for wasn't her idea of life. She tried to brush it off as a one-time event and settled back into her usual eighty- to ninety-hour week.

•   •   •

A few weeks later, Ninjja was getting ready to start 8:00 a.m. interviews of potential candidates when she suddenly felt that the world around her was in a spin. She grabbed the table nearby and made her way to the sofa. Every time she tried to get up, the same phenomenon occurred. Being interviewed by a dizzy interviewer hardly qualified as a motivational tool to attract new talent, so she decided to give it a pass.

She got on the phone to express her inability to make it. Her colleague at the other end of the line was clearly upset and had no sympathy for her plight. "It's too late now; I can't let you drop out! Our panel will be now incomplete...how will we manage the logistics?" were just some of the darts that he threw at her in the five-minute monologue. Ninjja could only manage a brief "Assume that I am dead" and hung up.

There was no respite in the next several hours. Such a crazy bout of dizziness was new to her, and she felt it was high time she visited a doctor. Fortunately, she hadn't needed to see a general physician since she had moved to this new city, but as her "good health" coupon seemed near expiry, she took a taxi to the doctor whom one of her colleagues recommended. The diagnosis was very intriguing.

"You are suffering from vertigo, which could be due to stress," the doctor announced. "Due to stress, sometimes a pressure imbalance occurs in the eardrums, which leads to vertigo."

"But how can I be stressed? I really enjoy the work I do...so what's wrong if I end up working long hours?" Ninjja tried to argue.

The doctor was kind enough to continue the conversation. He explained, "Being upset, angry, or unhappy are not the only things that cause stress. If you are constantly pressed for time or you are trying to pack too many things in a short period, your system is bound to feel the tension, and it starts manifesting itself in many ways. Headaches, lower back pain, sleep deprivation, and dizziness are some of the early manifestations. If left unchecked, it can be a big killer. It can lead to serious physical illnesses like stomach ulcers, IBS, depression, heart disease, and so on." He stopped for a breath and gave her a pitying gaze. Ninjja gulped as she absorbed the information overload.

Ninjja had experienced emotional stress before, but this was something new. She was glad that she had discovered this before it was too late. The doctor comforted her that there was no reason to worry, but lifestyle changes would be necessary. Soon she was back to normal, but she knew that it was time to take stock of her habits and lifestyle yet again. She was happy to see a young doctor from the clan of "Doxtinct", but suspected a strong rebuttal from "SOULMAC".

Previous wake-up calls had helped her in controlling her eating habits, including some form of exercise in her routine, and forced her to follow a tighter project management (which, in turn, helped with time management). The new wake-up call forced her to relook at her calendar with a fine comb. Did she really need to attend so many conferences? Did she really need to sign up for so many additional office responsibilities? The list was definitely not short. As Ninjja was going to bed that night, she was feeling much lighter, and Arv's comment reverberated in her mind—"Get a grip on your life, Ninjja." She vowed to call him the next day and made a small note for herself in the little yellow diary.

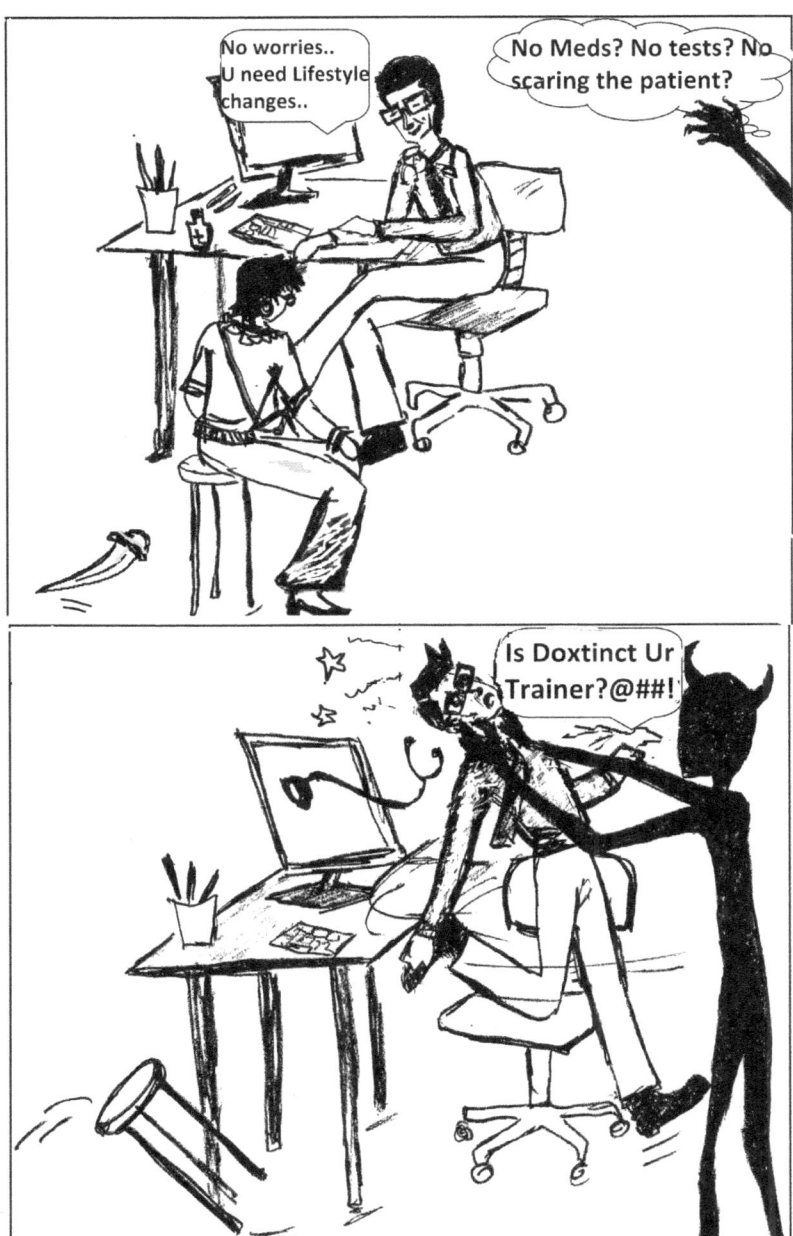

Ninjja suffers from vertigo

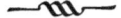

My Survival Mantra

1. Don't assume that your regular physician will always know what is right for you.
2. When in doubt, seek a second opinion.
3. Always have health insurance and carefully select the plan.
4. Don't rush to a specialist based on your perceived issue.
5. Overseas insurance is not a blank check.
6. A balanced lifestyle holds the secret of many a cure.
7. In emergency situations (e.g., an accident), don't run to the closest hospital.
8. **Several diseases (like ulcers, insomnia, heart disease, etc.) may have stress as the underlying cause.** Make sure that this link is not ignored while deciding on the treatment. That stress is due only to "emotional reasons" is a myth. Your work and lifestyle can also be a big contributor. Learn to read the symptoms of stress (like lower back pain, headaches, indigestion, dizziness, etc.) and take stock of your working habits. You are the one who is best positioned to unearth potential sources of stress and then reduce the clutter. Techniques like yoga and meditation can help, but ultimately it is your mindset and attitude that you need to master.

NOVEMBER 2006

The recent wake-up call and calming influence from Arv had made Ninjja much more relaxed in her approach to work and life. She was gradually learning the art of distinguishing "critical" from "good to have". She also discovered the therapeutic effects of saying no once in a while, and she was more aware and comfortable with making difficult choices at work and living with the implications of her choices. Overall, her status could be defined as "content with life."

To take her happiness quotient to a different level, she received two "good news" calls in quick succession. Her sister was expecting her first child—a baby girl—and her long-lost friend was moving back to India for an assignment.

She couldn't believe that soon she would become an aunt! She really wished she had wings so that she could share her joy with every living being on the planet.

The work suddenly started appearing super easy. The happy feeling that had enveloped her acted as an analgesic for some of the unproductive meetings she had to participate in.

As luck would have it, she received an invitation for a conference in the United States for the coming month. There was no way this was going into her "deprioritize bucket" this time. The countdown had begun! To celebrate, Ninjja ordered a full-blown Indian thali replete with starters, rich gravies, and desserts.

• • •

The food was a delight while it lasted, but the night that followed was a hell that Ninjja wouldn't forget all her life.

. . .

She had fallen asleep very quickly, but some discomfort kept her tossing and turning. Within a few hours, she knew what was happening: full-blown hives had erupted with uncontrollable itching. Possibly, some mushrooms (which she was allergic to) had accidentally found their way into her mixed-vegetables dish (where different ingredients are difficult to identify in any case).

Ninjja had never experienced anything so severe before. Unfortunately, the hotel didn't have any antiallergy medicine in stock. The only thing that Ninjja could do in the meanwhile was to kick herself for not keeping a pill handy with her. It took the hotel almost three hours to procure something in the middle of the night.

The medicine finally put her to sleep again. After a few hours, when she woke up, the hives were still there! In addition, she felt a lump in her throat and found it hard to speak and breathe. It was only six o'clock in the morning, and there was no way she could see a doctor at that hour. In that moment of distress, she thought of calling a doctor that her company had recently enrolled to help out employees with their health-care issues. Ninjja decided to take her chances.

Fortunately, the doctor promptly took her call, and within two minutes of hearing her symptoms, he asked her to rush to the emergency room.

. . .

When she reached the hospital, the doctor on duty in the emergency ward was ready to receive her. After two strong dosages of steroidal injections, she could feel her voice and breath coming back. Apparently, the allergy was so severe that it had started choking her windpipe. A delay would have meant a life-threatening situation. She was asked to stay under observation for at least twenty-four hours, which seemed reasonable.

The doctor also used his influence to get her a bed (albeit in a maternity ward!), which was a big achievement given the shortage level. A few hours later, the expert also paid a visit to determine whether the line of treatment required any changes. This was Ninjja's first experience of being alone in the hospital for twenty-four hours.

As she lay there with drips and some other paraphernalia attached to her arms, she didn't know what she would have done without the guidance from her company doctor. He had added tremendous value on two counts:

1) Reading symptoms right and creating a sense of urgency in the patient for an illness that usually falls in the "nonthreatening" category.
2) Taking her call at an odd hour and navigating through the treatment process, including emergency attention, expert input, and even the admission process.

She was fortunate enough to work for a firm that cared enough and had the means to afford a high-quality doctor. To serve the broader population with the same personalized attention, even within the corporate world, would be a Herculean task. The economics as well as the feasibility of getting so many doctors spread across different locations would be a killer. There was a need to think outside of the box to create an alternate model that was not dependent on the benevolence of the employing company. The idea of building a "health-care navigator" had starting forming in her mind when the attendant arrived with a fairly unattractive food serving.

She decided to ignore her taste buds and gulp down the calories that the steroids in her body were desperately demanding. She had barely finished the sweet pudding, in the hope of recovering from the aftertaste of the insipid meal that she had just devoured, when the nurse arrived with a syringe. "I need to draw a blood sample," she announced. Ninjja dutifully informed the nurse that she had just had a meal, including desserts, and hoped that it wouldn't interfere with the test results. The nurse nodded (whether it was a yes or a no wasn't entirely clear) and poked in the needle.

The combination of antihistamines, steroids and food had magnified the effect of gravity at least ten times, and Ninjja slipped into another bout of deep slumber. The synchronized howling of babies brought her back to the current world. It took her five minutes to become aware of the surroundings and be reminded that she was recovering from her allergies in a maternity ward.

Soon, the nurse was back with more medicines and test reports. "Your blood sugar is high. Everything else is normal. I will check with doctor regarding additional medication," she informed Ninjja in an attempt to be helpful. Despite feeling very heavy, Ninjja's eyes popped out, and she started wondering if she had become so dull that she was hallucinating—or was this indeed "NurSpOilymaking a reappearance?

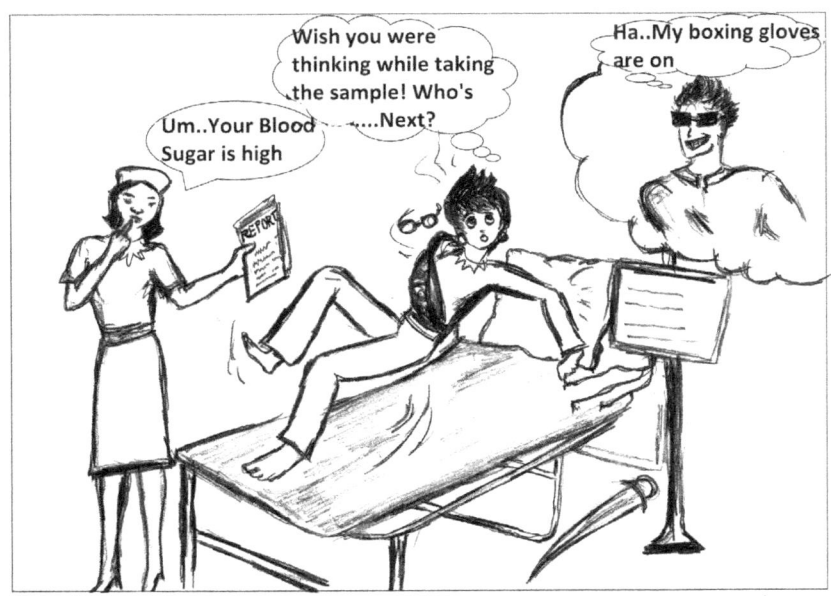

Ninjja encounters NurSpOily

Later in the evening, the doctor emerged again and was clever enough to dismiss the blood-sugar issue as something insignificant "This could also be due to steroids or due to food…you can do a fasting test when convenient." *If the test was going to be inconclusive, why was it done in the first place?* Ninjja wondered, but she didn't have the courage to ask, given that the doctor had already been very helpful. To console herself, she thought that maybe the hospitals loved to do additional analyses, as was the case in her profession, where innumerable hours got spent in doing analyses that the client had never asked for but that their firm's own "high bar for truth" compelled them to do. The only difference was that the clients never paid for the additional analyses in her profession!

• • •

Despite all the help from the doctor, the discharge process remained a draconian, time-consuming process. Fortunately, her colleagues, who had come to check on her, ended up bearing the brunt of the paperwork that followed, and they heaved a sigh of relief when they were finally out in the open air. "Why can't this be a smooth and pleasant checkout experience, as one has in good hotels?" one of her colleagues commented wryly, inviting chuckles from the others.

Ninjja absorbed it silently and felt that the comment wasn't without merit.

. . .

DECEMBER 2006

It was a chilly morning, and Ninjja reluctantly pulled herself out of the comfort of her cozy bed to catch a 6:30 a.m. flight. The phenomenon of recalcitrant trousers had struck again—thanks to the side effect of weight gain due to steroids. A quarter to five in the morning was not the time she wanted to have a fight with her trousers. With a heavy heart, she settled for an Indian dress, which has the capability of hiding an ever-growing body mass.

She vowed to go on a vegetables-and-fruit diet, at least for dinners. She was determined to avoid investing in a fresh set of clothes. Under the added pressure of potential snide comments from her friend Amit, whom she was planning to meet for dinner that day, she decided to skip breakfast on the flight.

After the usual rituals of "Sorry for the delay, which was beyond our control" and "Tighten your seat belt," the plane started its pushback, and Ninjja settled down for a nap. She was woken up by something that sounded like an argument between her copassenger and the flight attendant. Her fellow passenger was miffed that the vegetarian menu was loaded with mushrooms, which he was allergic to.

That was enough to get Ninjja to fully awaken and actively participate in a diatribe against mushrooms and the poor judgment that the airline displayed in selecting the menu. Unfortunately, the flight attendant had to bear the brunt of this anger for no fault of hers. Alas, such is life!

On the positive side, there was a sudden connection with her copassenger, which started a spontaneous, free flow of experiences and stories covering a very wide range of topics. The discussion started with the lack of sensitivity to allergies that one sees in the hospitality industry and then meandered around work-life balance, uncompetitive salaries in government, health-care challenges, and more. That they managed such smooth transitions between such diverse topics was a pleasant surprise for Ninjja, who was used to sticking to a framework or a structure during the course of her work. Today, following the course of nature (which doesn't follow a predefined structure or an agenda) allowed her a glimpse of so many different facets of life.

One such story that her copassenger narrated was that of a young girl who was suffering from a strange disease.

This young girl, who was just twenty-one years of age, had a serious issue with bone degradation. Her bones were aging much faster than normal, and she was told that she should be mentally prepared to have a curved back and the body of a sixty-year-old at thirty. She was warned that having a normal married life with children was something she shouldn't imagine even in her dreams. If she survived beyond age forty, she would have to lead the life of a cripple. This

was a horrible discovery for someone who had just started exploring life. She had the zest to enjoy life to the fullest, and her parents
didn't want to give up. All the possible top-notch institutions, unfortunately, gave them the same answer.

Not willing to let go, they kept trying whatever alternate therapies their family and friends popped at them. Needless to say, even
with this Herculean effort, there were no signs of improvement.
During one such sympathetic conversation at a gathering, they heard
about an institute located in southern India that practiced traditional
Ayurvedic medicine and ancient healing techniques of India. This institute had a few nuggets to its credit of curing untreatable diseases.
With no other option in sight, they decided to undertake the thirty-
six-hour journey, though not expecting much to come out of it.

After the initial review, they were told that there was a ray of
hope, but it would require a strict regimen and a stay at the institute
for two months. Given that all the other doors were closed, they conceded. Indeed, the regimen was tough, with dictates on what, when,
and how much to eat, along with medicines and other therapies.
Such was the desperation of the family that they happily complied
with every minute instruction.

Contrary to their initial expectations, there was a surprising improvement by the end of two months. The girl herself couldn't believe what she saw. Finally, she was allowed to get back to her home
and was given strict lifestyle guidelines to maintain her health. She
was also supposed to go back for a checkup after six months and repeat the treatment every two to three years. The young girl treated
this as her holy grail and continued to reap the benefits.

Ten years later, the same young girl, now a married woman with a
child, was still going strong, had a job, and walked with a straight back!

• • •

The story of the young girl left a lasting impression on Ninjja. She kicked herself for not making a note of the specifics that could be shared more broadly for the benefit of others in similar situation. However, one thing was clear. Alternative medicines and treatments could be very powerful—provided one knew the right source! There was a high proportion of quacks in the alternative-medicine profession, but if one knew where to look, there was hope. Information asymmetry was the biggest impediment.

The other challenge that this example showed her was that alternate therapies were often resorted to when there was no hope left through the conventional route, making it difficult for their stats to look good. Ninjja also wondered, if the choice was between getting a quick remedy without following strict dietary and lifestyle changes and spending several months for a cure (in some cases actually taking time off from work), what would one prefer? Ninjja wasn't sure which option she would choose unless the situation actually pushed her to the wall.

She also noted this down as a challenge of the health-care system for future reference.

A receiver's perspective on health-care challenges

1. Death of the quintessential family doctor
2. Moral corruption spreading its wings in the medical profession
3. Affordability of health care

4. Quality of attendants and nurses

5. **Availability and credibility of information on alternate cures**: Homeopathy, Ayurveda, and other alternate cures have long enjoyed the status of poor and fraudulent cousins of allopathic treatment, thanks to the less stringent regulatory mechanisms, low earning potential, and unscrupulous quacks. At the same time, many people have a "miracle story" of someone who got cured through these alternate routes. This route is conveniently forgotten for inherent lack of trust, time taken for healing, difficult lifestyle changes, and so on, till one is pushed to the wall. Given the holistic curing potential that these alternatives offer, it is surprising that even in the information age, we don't have a mechanism of converting this word of mouth to a systematic, credible source of information. A google search for "best homeopaths" reveals many such doctors (independently or collectively) boasting of their success, along with testimonials from the purported patients. Wouldn't it be valuable if there were a mechanism to verify the credibility of online claims as well as share information about unsung heroes who have cured many but have only a narrow sphere of influence limited by the range of word of mouth?

—ɯ—

. . .

MARCH 2007

Finally, the day that Ninjja was waiting for had arrived. She was flying off to the United States to meet her sister and share the joy of the new life taking shape inside her. She had to work very hard to contain her excitement and focus her energy on the content of the conference and networking—both of which were important for her career. The two days seemed very long; and finally, when her three-day break to visit her sister started, the days seemed to evaporate rather quickly.

In a jiffy she was back to her routine. But the countdown to the day of baby's arrival had begun.

. . .

Four

The Flight

JUNE 2007

Ninjja's parents had already arrived at their base station (Ninjja's home) to take their flight to the United States. Preparations were in full swing, with daily shopping sprees that were getting more difficult by the day. The maximum baggage allowance of the airlines wasn't enough to contain all the goodies that they wanted to take for their yet-to-arrive first granddaughter. The countdown was already on, with just one day to go before the flight. After all the suitcases were packed with highest efficiency, some empty space still remained.

It would have been sacrilege to let it go to waste, so Ninjja and her mom decided to make another trip to a nearby mall, while her dad chose to stay home instead. Later on, that would prove to be a wise decision.

• • •

As the rickshaw reached the mall, the novice driver couldn't control his speed and couldn't judge the terrain, which was brilliantly dug up to make way for a metro line. As always, there was no signage to warn the unsuspecting and inexperienced drivers (who existed in abundance). Before the driver could act on Ninjja's screams of "Slow down, there is a ditch!" one front tire and one back tire had landed in the ditch, and the vehicle was ready to topple over. Ninjja was not agile enough to do something in the next few seconds, and she came back to reality only after hearing her mother scream in pain.

Ninjja found her feet quickly, and with the help of the crowd that had quickly gathered, she tried to lift her mother out of the ditch. The difficulty that her mother had in standing indicated that she might require a hospital visit. As always, people muttered several names of hospitals, and fortunately Ninjja remembered her previous lesson of being diligent when choosing a hospital. One of the names that was mentioned had a good reputation, and Ninjja decided to make it their next destination.

The emergency machinery was effective and sprang into action in no time. Ninjja had a sense of déjà vu as the X-ray was being taken. The doctor on duty reviewed the X-ray and announced, "Congratulations, there is no fracture. You can go home and rest." However, the level of immobility and the degree of pain signified that something was amiss. Ninjja decided to request for a specialist consultation.

Half an hour later, when the specialist arrived, he inspired a sense of confidence with his dexterity in the physical examination. His annoyance with the doctor on emergency duty was apparent as he started educating him on how to read fine hairline fractures in an X-ray.

The next course of action was a no-brainer. Given that the fracture was in the waist, staying flat on the bed was the only option.

Managing the hospital logistics seemed easier compared to the task at hand—changing flight logistics and breaking the bad news to her sister!

After going through the motions, when Ninjja finally settled down, she couldn't help wondering about the coincidence of experience with doctors on emergency duty. Are they the worst lot, or are they still in training? Is there no difference between an average hospital and a renowned hospital? On deeper reflection, she took solace in the fact that there was a big difference in the skill level of the orthopedic specialist. The consequences of improper diagnosis (as in case of the fracture she had suffered earlier that went undetected even by the specialist) could have been detrimental for someone much older. She thanked her stars for being able to implement her learning and hoped for the best. She started flipping through her yellow diary and felt there was a need to refine her previous lesson regarding hospital visits after an accident. She tried to squeeze one sentence in the available space.

My Survival Mantra

7. In situations of emergency (e.g., an accident), don't run to the closest hospital...If you are unsure regarding the advice of the doctor on emergency duty, it might be worthwhile to demand a specialist for consultation. This is especially relevant in developing countries like India where emergency services like 911 are primitive.

Ninjja was dumbfounded by the fragility of life that this incident showed her. In less than a minute, three things had changed dramatically for her mother:

- Position: from being hyperactive to being tied to her bed.
- Geography: Delhi instead of San Francisco (where she would have been in forty-eight hours).
- State of mind: from overexcitement to utter despair.

The helplessness that her sister felt compounded the unnerving effect. "There couldn't have been a worse moment for this accident," Ninjja said to herself, wondering if she was gifted with a uniquely accident-prone family. She consoled herself by thinking about some other people she knew who had a more scintillating track record.

Ninjja's work schedule was wrecked with commuting between the hospital, home, and her workplace and being on phone calls with her concerned sister and brother-in-law. Five days had gone by, and Ninjja's observation of activities at the hospital didn't indicate that anything significant was being done. Finally, she couldn't control her urge to discuss this with the doctor. "Doctor, can't I take her home and get a nurse to give her the injections? In the best-case scenario, it would be three weeks before she can move about. I can't do this for so long…we would be a lot more comfortable…emotionally and physically, as well as financially, if we could be at home…"

The doctor's response completely surprised her. "Sure, she can be discharged anytime." He continued, "But won't you be better off on costs and comfort by staying at the hospital? Anyway, your employer or the insurance company will reimburse the claim." The statement left Ninjja gasping for breath. She gathered herself and informed the doctor of their situation regarding the insurance policy.

To limit the financial damage that was about to hit Ninjja, he started the discharge formalities immediately. Ninjja thanked the doctor and proceeded to the billing desk while her parents waited for the ambulance to get ready. The bill came to a whopping Rs. 50,000 (~US$1,000), with a liberal sprinkling of visits from multiple doctors that varied from five to fifteen minutes. Ninjja was in a state of shock at the bill amount for a situation that required only a doctor's expertise for diagnosis and advice on painkillers while nature took its course for healing. At best, her mind could justify one or two days for the hospital stay to manage the pain and observe for any unforeseen complications. Her mother might have exceeded the hospital stay required for heart surgery in the United States (which was four to seven days) if she hadn't intervened!

. . .

The ambulance staff was in a big hurry and was oblivious to the fact that they were carrying an immobile human being on the stretcher and not lifeless goods. A few mercy pleas and screams later, Ninjja and her mother got settled in the vehicle and were glad to be getting home. The same process of screaming was repeated before Ninjja's mother found herself in the comfort of her own bed. Ninjja's expectations of better end-to-end service, at least from a premium hospital, crashed to the ground. She consoled herself with the fact that they had received the correct diagnosis and were discharged without any fuss once she raised the issue.

As her stress eased a bit, the bigger issue that had escaped her so far came back with an enormity that dwarfed everything else that had rattled her nerves: *Why should the length of a hospital stay or the intensity of treatment that one receives depend on whether one has an employer reimbursing the bill or has an insurance company to back it up?* Logic refused to accept any linkage between the two. The implicit dependence that seemed to have gotten established had several repercussions. She made a mental note of the top three that struck her:

1) **Act as a deterrent to people without the luxury of reimbursement**:
   The assumption of the premium hospitals that any patient walking in has an employer who will reimburse the costs or has insurance generous enough to cover all the hospitalization charges would either leave patients with sticker shock or completely deter them. Although the hospitals could earn supernormal profits on some patients, they would also lose a significant share of other potential customers who could have visited otherwise.

2) **Increase the financial burden on corporate employers or the insurance provider,** impacting their willingness to provide such services. An employer who made provisions to take care of the health of its employees would have done so in good faith. *Shouldn't unscrupulous use of that facility by the hospitals, either alone or in connivance with the patients, be considered a breach of trust and dealt with accordingly?* If the abuse of such benefits went too far, it would not be surprising if the employers chose to withdraw such facilities or structured a deal to pass on the risks. In an economy where less than 15 percent of people have some sort of medical coverage, such a trend could be catastrophic to the desired aggressive growth in medical coverage.

3) **Subject patients to higher long-term risks** of being administered more costly and higher-intensity medicines and procedures when something simpler could have worked better.

Ninjja tried to step into the shoes of patients who had full medical coverage and visualized a situation when the patient is presented with a choice of going for a more expensive treatment. *If I were on a shopping treat, and someone else were going to pay the full bill, I might go for the most expensive stuff that I like*, Ninjja thought. *Why wouldn't the same apply to a patient, if he or she is not aware of the associated downside or long-term risks? Are all those angioplasties really required?* She wasn't sure now. She remembered the case of her neighbor, whose dad was admitted to the hospital for some chest pain. While the family had stepped out, the doctors had a little chat with the old man and learned that his employer gave him health coverage. By the time her neighbor came back to the hospital, the surgery was done, and the dad was happily recovering. Since the dad was doing fine and there was no financial damage that the neighbor's family had to wrestle with, they happily thanked the doctors and forgot about the whole episode. The more Ninjja thought about it, the scarier it felt. *What percentage of surgeries in the private hospitals are unnecessary?* Ninjja wondered if employees with full health coverage from their employers (e.g., government employees) had a higher share of doctor's visits and went through more intensive procedures.

To make more informed and appropriate decisions, there was a need to share the pain across all parties. The interim opportunities of extracting more money from a patient would not be a strategy that could continue to win in the long term. She thought of summarizing this new challenge that she had discovered in her diary.

—⚏—

A receiver's perspective on health-care challenges

1) Death of the quintessential family doctor
2) Moral corruption spreading its wings in the medical profession
3) Affordability of health care
4) Quality of attendants and nurses
5) Availability and credibility of information on alternative cures
6) **Indiscreet use and abuse of health-care reimbursements and insurance**: Sometimes, short-term gains taint the judgment of health-care providers. The lack of a system to align everyone's goals toward the most efficient mode of treatment creates divergent motives. A tendency to consider it as a win-win situation for the patient and the hospitals when the actual cost is borne by either the employer or the insurance company could be detrimental to patients' long-term health and can dig a bigger hole in the pocket of the provider than it should. In a country with such a low penetration of health coverage (either through employers or through insurance providers), such behavior could deter the aggressive growth of health coverage and further aggravate the

challenges. Perhaps it is time to pause and make corrections-before it is too late! Sharing financial pain (e.g., through deductibles where the patient bears a small portion of costs) and tighter vigilance and penalties for hospitals that breach the trust placed in them might be a good place to start.

—ↄↄↄ—

. . .

Everyone in Ninjja's household had settled into the new routine of not seeing her mother scamper around the house and keep everything in order. A new maid had come in as a savior, and Ninjja's father, who was normally the one being taken care of, had suddenly emerged as the knight in shining armor. His willpower to rise to the need of the hour compensated for his otherwise delicate physical health. Her mother had started devouring books when she got bored with flipping through TV channels and was trying hard to keep her mind off her fate of not being able to hold her grandchild in the first few hours after birth.

Ninjja was amazed to see the flexibility with which humans were able to settle into a new, steady state.

. . .

One month went by rather slowly. The doctor was nice enough to make home visits and provided the much-needed assurance that he was able to see signs of improvement, though none of this was visible to Ninjja or to her dad.

JULY 31, 2007

Finally, the much-awaited visible improvements appeared: Ninjja's mother was able to move a few feet with the help of a walker.

To celebrate the occasion, they had a hearty meal and huddled together to flip through channels on TV as their group activity. The consensus on which program could be watched for the next ten minutes had just begun to emerge when the telephone rang. It was Ninjja's brother-in-law, Kuru, calling from the hospital. He cheerfully informed them that the baby might arrive anytime now. "What? Isn't the due date still a few days away?" Ninjja asked in a perplexed tone.

"Well, there was some goof-up at the doctor's end. When we came today for the regular checkup, the OB/GYN informed us that she had miscalculated the date. Actually, the baby is overdue. The doctor is doing a cesarean operation while we speak. There are no complications, so just relax," he responded calmly.

Three of them tried to participate in Kuru's exuberance and carefully shielded any signs of anxiety from showing. He had to hang up, as the nurse was calling him.

Ninjja had no experience in this area, so she turned to her mother to check if doctors often miscalculated the due date. A few minutes later, the phone rang again. This time Ninjja heard a baby cry as though she were trying to test the full potential of her lungs. Ninjja was so ecstatic that she forgot to switch to speaker mode. Fortunately, the baby was in no mood to rest anytime soon, so the grandparents could get their fill of joy. The crying felt like music to their ears and pumped enough energy into Ninjja's mother's atrophied limbs for her to get up from the bed.

The day could not have ended any better for Ninjja and her family.

. . .

Two days later, Ninjja's sister had recovered from the drowsiness induced by the anesthesia and was ready to be discharged from the hospital. She was quite irritable and was missing her parents terribly. Fortunately, her friends had all stepped up to the occasion and gone all out to make her feel completely pampered. Ninjja's mother could not control her urge to provide long-distance advice on what to eat, what to avoid, and a very long list of dos and don'ts. Ninjja was sometimes surprised to hear her sister's irritated tone and her lack of chattiness, which was very much unlike her. Kuru came in her sister's defense and explained the concept of "postpartum depression" to Ninjja. "Yeah, whatever! As long as you are happy with the situation, I am fine." Ninjja chose to ignore this issue.

. . .

Ninjja's mother was making speedy progress now. A few feet of movement became a few meters of movement, and now she was advised to walk around in the house two or three times a day with the support of a walker. However, the doctor was still unwilling to commit to a date when she would be fit enough for long-distance air travel. But the situation was comfortable enough for Ninjja to resume her normal work style, which was to work from the client's location. The sight of her parents waving to her from the balcony with beaming smiles was enough to energize her for the day and help her survive the uninspiring food that awaited her on the plane.

. . .

Ninjja was sitting on her bed in the hotel room, replying to social e-mails with the TV running in the background. She was hoping that the mind-numbing staged reality show running at that hour would help her relax.

Suddenly, a ring of her phone that felt unusually loud jerked her out to the real world. It was past midnight, and Ninjja somehow had a sinking feeling as she picked up the phone.

"How quickly can you come here? We need you…" That was Kuru's somber voice. Such a sudden and unusual request didn't help Ninjja's already agitated nerves. She felt a choking feeling in her throat as she mumbled, "What happened? Is everything all right?… Say something…don't scare me, please…" There was a thirty-second silence on the other end that felt like an eternity.

Then she heard his faint voice. "Your sister has suffered a brain hemorrhage. The neurosurgeon has just gone to see her. We don't know what the chances are…" His voice trailed off into sobbing.

Ninjja was numbed as though all the air around her had been sucked out. She felt that she was floating in a vacuum in a no-gravity zone. A few seconds later, the baby's wailing in the background got her back to the reality that was staring at them.

"Let me find the earliest flight that I can take," was all that she could manage to utter. She had no strength left to say a few words to inspire hope, as is typically done in such situations. After hanging up the phone, she started browsing desperately for flight options, while her brain was trying to concoct a believable enough story that she could use to convince her parents regarding her sudden trip to the United States. She wasn't sure what was going to be more difficult—telling the truth or watching her parents deal with it. So, she chose a third path—the easier path of concealing the reality.

. . .

Fifty restless hours later, she was finally sitting on a plane in a state of limbo. The status update on her sister before takeoff indicated "status quo," which did nothing to offer her respite. Just four months ago, she couldn't contain her excitement when she had boarded her US flight, and now, she was sitting there motionless, refusing to stir even after repeated requests by her fellow passenger, who deserved some courtesy to get to his window seat. "Are you all right?" Ninjja was being nudged by the flight attendant now.

The gentle prodding pulled Ninjja out of her reverie, and she bolted out of her seat, mumbling, "I am so sorry." Her despair still overruled the embarrassment she had just undergone, and Ninjja again relapsed into her spell.

Several hours later, her aching legs and sore back forced her to come out of her feeling of nothingness and acknowledge the state of her body. It was time to take some action. Ninjja started looking for the levers for the footrest, but there were none in this old plane. She decided to use her hand baggage as a substitute and reclined her seat by the few degrees that were possible. These incremental changes, however, didn't do much to soothe her aching body and agitated mind. *Maybe if I could watch some movies to distract my mind...*Ninjja said to herself, and she started looking for the personal screen. Alas, there was no such thing.

This European airline seemed to have a really clear business model. Based on the experience so far, Ninjja could see that they were in the business of transporting people from point A to point B in living condition. Anything beyond that, like physical comfort and entertainment, was clearly out of their scope. These specially designed economy seats, intended to pack as many people as possible, could barely accommodate Ninjja's body. Ninjja said a silent prayer for the people endowed with slightly heavier physical form and tried to divert her mind by reading some worthy articles stored on her laptop. Ninjja read every word very carefully, but somehow she was having difficulty in registering whole sentences. She didn't want to give up and kept going through the pages line by line. While the process didn't result in any better comprehension of the esoteric topic of climate change, it surely helped her in killing some time. Ninjja knew that comprehending anything required coordinated effort between mind and body, but this was the first time that this concept had come to life for her. She was now fully aware that her mind and body were no longer working as a team. Tired with the struggle of the last few hours and taking cues from the low-battery alarm on her laptop, she closed her eyes and waited for the flight to land in Europe.

As the confluence of all the negative forces would have it, the delayed arrival didn't leave Ninjja with any time to make the required phone call to check on her sister. She barely scraped through the elaborate security and transit procedures to land at her seat in a huff.

The unknown can sometimes torment one even more than the knowledge of a gruesome truth. Unfortunately, Ninjja had no option but to deal with the unknown for the next nine hours.

. . .

The time went by rather slowly. When the landing announcement struck her ears, it felt like she had been in the plane for eternity. It was time to pull herself together and join the flow of people. Ninjja thanked the San Francisco airport for consistently giving her the same smooth exit experience that she couldn't have wanted more than in this current trip. As she was wheeling her small bag toward the exit, she saw a young man waving at her. Ninjja looked carefully, and with some mental effort, she remembered him as a friend of her sister's, whose pictures she had seen in several albums. He came forward after seeing Ninjja demonstrate some signs of recognition and took her bag. He informed Ninjja that her sister was responding well to the treatment, and the doctors were hopeful that she might not need neurosurgery.

After twenty-four hours of agony, this piece of news acted as a relaxing music for Ninjja's overstressed brain and nerves. She took in a deep breath for her oxygen-starved lungs and found the energy to inquire about the baby. She was also filled with a sense of guilt for really not thinking about the baby in the past seventy-five hours.

The little one wouldn't have gotten much attention and care at all. Ninjja was really desperate to see both the mother and the child and wished that she could again fly. In this one-hour drive, she felt the existence of all the thirty-six hundred seconds that passed. She learned that a distant cousin had offered to take care of the baby while Kuru spent his days and nights at the hospital waiting for some good news. She silently thanked this savior cousin of hers, whose existence was unknown to her till this very moment.

· · ·

Finally, the moment of truth arrived. She was standing face-to-face with her sister in the ICU, who gave her the best cheerful smile that was possible in her current feeble state. Ninjja gently stroked her hair for want of words and tried to hide her nervousness, which was aggravated by a variety of devices attached to her sister's body.

Ninjja was desperate to find any signals of hope and was glad to find some that she could hang on to for support. Focusing on the positives helped her ward off the depressing thoughts. She was surprised to hear her own voice as she uttered, "You will be back home soon." For a split second, a shadow of gloom passed through her sister's face as she spoke in a muffled tone. "I have noises in my head, and...I can't see you properly." Before Ninjja could react and ask any further questions, an attendant politely informed her that it was time to leave the patient alone to recuperate.

As Ninjja stepped out, her sister's words were still ringing in her head. Ninjja tried to reconcile with the fact that the tug-of-war between hope and despair was going to go on for some more time, but it wasn't easy. Ninjja looked around, but she saw no doctor available. She could see a nurses' station at the far end of the corridor and rushed toward it. "Hi, I want to talk about the patient in room number three. Can you please help?" she blurted out as soon as she had the attention of the nurse manning the station. "I am her sister. She can't see properly...and in her head..."

Ninjja didn't need to expend her energy any further as the nurse cut her off in a calm voice, "Yes, I know. Look, dear," she continued, "the stroke has hit her in the lower part of her brain, which has affected the nerves responsible for vision. You are lucky. She got here just in time. Don't you worry! She is a brave girl."

The bullish sentiment expressed by the nurse didn't exactly lift Ninjja's spirits, nor did it give any more clarity on her sister's chance of recovery. The nurse carefully chose the path of "no comments or talk to the doctor" for any further questions related to the outlook on the patient's recovery. The only comfort that Ninjja could draw from this conversation was that the ground staff was fully aware of the condition of the patient and that her sister had made it to the hospital in time (within three hours after the stroke) to have a chance of survival. Ninjja now started her wait for the next milestone—the doctor's visit—and hoped that she would get some information, at least on what lay ahead. Her thoughts drifted toward her little niece, and she wondered if the baby had any idea of where her mother was and the state that she was in. Ninjja came back to reality as the nurse informed her that Kuru was waiting for her downstairs in the parking lot.

Ninjja started descending the stairs, not fully clear about the instruction and perplexed that her brother-in-law chose not to come inside the hospital. The parking lot was a short walk from the entrance, and without any extra effort, she managed to spot Kuru waiting outside the familiar Honda Civic. He looked fairly composed despite the current circumstances, and waved at her. Even before she could speak, he read the question running through her mind and said, "Doctors don't recommend bringing infants to the hospital for fear of infections. I have picked up Ira from your cousin's home, so I couldn't come upstairs."

Now the mystery was beginning to clear, but Ninjja didn't see anyone else around who would have carried and managed the infant during the two-hour drive. "Don't you want to see Ira?" Kuru asked, reading the confusion on her face as he opened the back door. Ninjja peeped inside and was awestruck by the sight of a tiny infant sleeping blissfully in the car seat. She looked so serene that, for a moment, Ninjja forgot all the turbulence that had afflicted her for the past few days.

"Wow, she is so small...I have never seen a human this size in my entire life," Ninjja exclaimed. She was also amazed to see the way

Kuru went about handling the tiny infant all by himself effortlessly. Possibly the environment that he was living in had given him the confidence to manage most situations independently. Back home, a two-hour drive with a seven-day-old infant would have qualified for an entourage of family and domestic helpers—their numbers being sufficient to fill all the available space in the car (including the nonexistent spot for the infant's car seat).

For once, Ninjja noticed that it was possible for a society to manage with less through simplification, confidence, and good systems.

The ride home was short and peaceful as the infant decided to continue with her deep sleep. Once home, Kuru gave her a quick five minutes of instruction on "infant handling" and on the process of making bottled milk before he stepped out for a critical errand, promising to be back in fifteen minutes. Once she had shut the door, a panic attack engulfed her.

What if the baby decides to wake up?

· · ·

Sure enough, her hunch was right—within five minutes she was jolted off of the sofa by a deafening cry. The infant wanted to make sure she was heard loud and clear and was possibly testing the full capacity of her lungs and vocal chords.

Ninjja scampered to pick up the baby from her stroller and was terrified to see the amount of tears and redness of the infant's face. When two minutes of cuddling and comforting didn't yield any result, Ninjja went for the second and only other weapon left with her—milk.

She had to deposit the howling little monster back in her stroller to take care of the operations of making milk. Ninjja tried to remember the instructions and started mixing warm water with the formula with her trembling hands. The infant showed no signs of relenting and continued her rhythmic cry. Finally, three more minutes later, Ninjja gently picked up the infant again, cradled her at the angle that Kuru had advised, and hoped that the bottle of milk would act as the magic potion. As the decibel level of the infant's screams started dropping exponentially, Ninjja's fear gradually gave way to wonder and awe. "How does this tiny eight-pound form get this kind of energy and perseverance to go on this loudly for five straight minutes?" she was mumbling to herself when she heard Kuru turning the door handle. Ninjja was relieved to see him, but her sense of comfort was short-lived. Kuru offered some additional guidance regarding changing diapers and said that this time he would be gone for at least two hours. Meeting the doctor and visiting her sister couldn't possibly take less time. Ninjja could see the rationale, but she couldn't stop extrapolating the experience of the past fifteen minutes to the coming two hours. She was shuddering inside as Kuru opened the door. As though reading her mind, he said, "Don't you worry; she sleeps most of the time anyway," and shut the door behind him.

"Yeah, right!" said Ninjja as she turned around to look at the infant, who had now morphed into a complete symbol of tranquility. A few moments of peace turned her thoughts back to her sister, and she hoped to get some good news from the hospital upon Kuru's return.

The next two hours were uneventful. Kuru was back, and it was time for a shift change. Ninjja was going to spend the night at the hospital with her sister, while Kuru was going to be home with the baby. The only positive thing that Kuru had heard from the doctor was "She is stable; we are hopeful." This was better than nothing, and Ninjja entered the hospital this time with a more positive mind-set.

•   •   •

Ninjja could see that her sister was in terrible pain, despite a heavy dosage of painkillers. The nurse was happy to explain all the vitals being monitored and told Ninjja to be particularly careful about the blood-pressure alarm. Ninjja settled on the tiny, bench-like bed provided to her and started getting accustomed to the various ticking sounds and different lights from the monitors.

As the hours clicked by, Ninjja's eyelids started getting heavier, signaling an end to an unusually long day (factoring in the time difference). A loud alarm around two o'clock jolted her out of her catnap. The colored monitor showed that the systolic blood pressure was above 190, and Ninjja could see that her sister's expression was one of utter discomfort. In a state of panic, Ninjja ran outside to call in the nurse. The nurse was quick to respond and used an injection. Even after things appeared stable, Ninjja continued in her sitting position, not sure if she could declare victory.

Another interruption in the night came when her sister started complaining of unbearable pain in her legs. Ninjja knew that this was not a situation that demanded medicinal intervention and tried to help her with the old technique of gentle massage.

•   •   •

Daybreak brought the chirpy nurse back for her routine checkup on vitals and for administering the morning dose of medicines. Ninjja decided to take a walk to the cafetaria for a cup of coffee. She couldn't help noticing that all the nurses had smiles on their faces despite being in the stroke ward, where most patients were hanging between life and death or had a serious risk of lifelong impairment. The mood-lifting impact that the nurses' pleasant demeanor had on the patients and their attendants was anything but trivial.

Ninjja's own experiences back home with hospitals had involved a collection of sullen and stressed-out faces of medical staff, which accentuated the downward slope of one's emotional state. Ninjja wondered if this was due to the volume that the staff needed to handle back home—or was it due to a lack of behavioral training? Whatever the reason, there was a clear opportunity to improve on this dimension, with definite potential to have a positive impact on patients' health. As Ninjja walked back into the ward, she heard her sister complaining of a severe headache, and Ninjja overheard the nurse say, "OK...I will get Vy..." (that was the painkiller being administered).

A few hours went by, and Ninjja was glad that she was able to have at least some conversation (though sparingly) with her sister. A particularly poignant moment came when her sister entrusted her with few pages of scribbling that she had addressed to her newborn. "If I am not there, please give this letter to my baby when she grows up." She paused and continued, "Will you take care of her if something happens to me?" Ninjja tried her best to control the avalanche of tears and responded calmly, "Nothing is going to happen to you. You will read this letter to your daughter yourself and tell her the whole story when she grows up." She looked at her intently.

Then a friend dropped by, offering much-desired relief from a very emotional moment. He offered to drop Ninjja home and make way for Kuru to come back to the hospital. Ninjja walked out with a heavy heart and tried diverting her attention to the tiny companion that she was going to have with her for the rest of the day.

• • •

Once home, she was handed a thick parenting book and given a practical demonstration of wrapping up the baby like a bundle for additional protection. Ninjja could see that the infant had already started expressing her discontent with the arrangement and had managed to free up one of her hands from the soft blanket that was tying her down.

They exchanged some additional notes, and then Kuru was ready to leave. This time, his parting words offered Ninjja a little more comfort than they had the last time. "Call me anytime," Kuru said as he shut the door behind him. The baby was in a quiet mood, allowing Ninjja time to flip through the parenting book. Apparently, all the expectant parents were advised to attend certain core classes and read this book in preparation for the arrival of the new life.

Ninjja flipped through the pages on various reasons why a baby could cry. She got educated about the importance of helping the baby burp, among many other things. She then stumbled upon a phenomenon called "SID," which stood for "sudden infant death," and her heart skipped a beat.

The number of SIDs stood at a staggering two thousand in the United States (third leading cause of infant mortality), whereas she had never even heard about this concept back home. One of the ways to counter SID given in the book was to ensure that the baby felt secure and had human contact. *That should be easy*, thought Ninjja as she snuggled closer to the infant and gently put an arm around her.

She wasn't sure of the impact that her action had, but it sure made Ninjja feel more secure. As she read more, she learned that there were many others who didn't find it that easy to stay in close touch with the baby while sleeping—modern-day lifestyle choices got in the way. For once, Ninjja was happy that the grandmothers' ground rules—no travel, keeping the baby close to the parents at all times, disciplined eating, and so on—were still being grudgingly followed by most new mothers back home.

Wanting your own space is fair, but how much space does one need to say that it is enough? Are we crossing the line when we need to keep the infant in a separate room in order to have our own space?

This was another example of the colossal difference that small things could make to someone's well-being.

• • •

Scared by her discovery, Ninjja held the baby so close that she could feel her heartbeat loud and clear. It was so fast that it sent a shock wave again through her spine. Her instinct was to call up Kuru, but instead she decided to fall back on the book for some guidance. The book informed her that it was normal for infants to have a heart rate of 120 or more.

Relieved to know that there was no reason to worry, Ninjja was equally amazed at how little she knew about the early days of human life. Ninjja was gradually getting comfortable with the tiny human's company and the new routine that had started forming.

• • •

Limbo had become the normal state of affairs. However, every evening Ninjja hoped that Kuru would come back with some good news from the doctor, and finally it did come!

The doctors believed that Ninjja's sister was now in the safe zone, and in due course (which was going to be several months), her body would be able to absorb the blood released in the brain due to hemorrhage. The fact that there would not be any need for surgery, and that Ninjja's sister could be released from the hospital in few days, got them so euphoric that the upcoming challenges of rehabilitation for the coming year didn't catch their attention even for a moment.

Ninjja couldn't wait to run to her sister when the baby, who was oblivious to the events since its birth, decided to go on a crying spree, breaking up the party. "Don't you understand anything, you cute little nut?" Ninjja muttered to the baby as she picked her up. After Ninjja's trial-and-error attempts at satisfying the baby's undeclared need, it finally obliged by falling asleep again.

Over the next few days in the hospital, Ninjja noticed that every three to four hours, her sister would get into in a mixed state of frenzy and stupor, complaining about pain, and would scream, "I want Vy…I have pain." Ninjja found it rather odd that a person in acute pain would mention the name of the medicine first and complain about the pain later. There was no other way but to ask in case of doubt, so Ninjja voiced her concern to the head nurse. Fortunately, she was receptive and listened to Ninjja patiently.

"Maybe the patient is getting addicted to the medicine, as these drugs for acute pain have narcotics in them." Ninjja's eyes widened with surprise as the nurse continued, "We may have to change the medicine...let me discuss it with the doctor." Sure enough, an hour later, the nurse did come back with the changed medicine.

Ninjja was glad that she had voiced her concern and hadn't assumed that the attending medical staff was omniscient. At the same time, she was also thankful to the nurse for lending a receptive ear and then using her experience to form an initial assessment of the situation. However, somewhere in her mind, a debate had ensued—*What if I hadn't been vigilant in observing the strange behavior? What if I had been shy about speaking up? Shouldn't the hospital have warned the patient and the care giver of potential side effects? Is it even possible?*

One part of her brain believed that it should be possible to provide a list of things to watch out for in different situations, while the other portion, which was already terrified to see the heaps of paperwork that a legally driven health-care system demanded, wanted to believe otherwise. Ninjja's thoughts wandered to the incident of few days ago when the nurse had handed over a thin booklet for her sister to read and sign. The contents had a lot of legal jargon that basically covered the hospital's legal liabilities as well as informed the patient of various risks of stroke and asked him or her to nominate someone to make decisions on his or her behalf in case of cognitive failure.

While the contents might have been very easy for the author to write, they didn't seem so simple for the patient who had suffered a stroke a few days ago. Ninjja remembered how uncomfortable and distraught her sister had become while going through just the first few pages. She couldn't go on reading anymore and threw the booklet back at Ninjja, saying, "Please read this and tell me where to sign; I don't want to think about death right now." Ninjja had wondered at that time whether the legal necessities had taken the transparency too far, to the extent that it had taken over compassion.

Today, Ninjja was wondering if the same legal system would make it difficult to decipher transparency. Even if the hospital made an attempt to explain the side effects or created a watch list for typical situations, the language required to ensure that they didn't get on the unfriendly side of the law with pharmaceutical companies, insurance companies, and even the patients would be so complicated that it would be difficult for normal humans. She started having doubts about the feasibility of a checklist. Given the uniqueness of each human body, under no situation would it be possible to prepare a 100-percent accurate list of things to watch out for. *If only it were possible for hospitals to share this information in good faith without worrying about the lawsuits!*

At a minimum, some informal forum to learn from the experiences of other people would indeed be helpful, she thought, and she decided to rest her case. Again, her belief that there was no substitute for being vigilant had been reaffirmed.

The changed drug was doing its job, and Ninjja was glad to see that her sister was no longer displaying symptoms of an addict.

· · ·

Days and nights seemed to go in a continuum, breaking the notion that one needs to rest the body at night. Ninjja didn't see any visible improvements in her sister during this time, but the following day finally brought some good news.

Ninjja's sister had gone back to her somnolent state after breakfast when the nurse came in and announced, "We will be releasing the patient today in few hours. The doctor has just confirmed it to me over the phone."

One nurse gradually started detaching various medical devices from the patient's body, while the other got busy with preparing the discharge folder. As the time for release came closer, Ninjja's excitement kept on growing, while her sister seemed to get more and more anxious with every passing minute.

The nurse came in with one final dosage of medicines that were to be administered in the hospital and started explaining the routine of medicines, the frequency of checkups, and various other things. The blood-pressure medicine that was to be administered three times a day caught Ninjja's attention, and she asked, "This looks to be a strong dosage; do we need to measure BP and administer this accordingly?"

"No," the nurse replied, "this is absolutely critical...given the level of her blood pressure, you have to give this medicine as prescribed."

Ninjja was taken aback by her sister's panic-stricken shriek. "I don't want to go; I am scared."

Ninjja immediately placed an arm around her sister and gently asked, "What are you scared of? The doctor says you are doing fine."

There was a moment of silence, and then came the response: "I will die at home."

Ninjja wasn't prepared for this answer. She paused for few minutes to collect herself and then tried comforting her sister using a combination of logic and affection. It did not work! Her sister was now suffering from a full-blown panic attack. Now, it was Ninjja's turn to get scared. Looking at the fear on her sister's face, her shaking hands, and the way she was clutching the bed and saying, "How will we know if something is going wrong?" Ninjja could not continue with her sermons and was forced to pause. The pause helped her appreciate her sister's predicament and the fact that the fear wasn't ill founded. For the past fifteen days, her sister had been in an ICU with various monitors providing guidance on the course of treatment or on emergency interventions. There were experienced nurses 24-7 on duty to take care of her. This was her comfort zone, and suddenly everything was being taken away in one shot.

Ninjja was now convinced that the transition needed to be more gradual, and she turned to talk to the nurse. "Why don't we let her stay at the hospital for one extra day without the monitors, so that she gets the comfort that she would be fine without them?" The nurse was unmoved as she retorted, "That won't be possible; the doctor says it is OK for her to go home."

"Well, then I would like to explain the situation to the doctor and seek his help." Ninjja's tone was genuine.

"Sorry, you won't be able to speak to the doctor; he won't be coming in today, as it is a Sunday."

Giving up easily wasn't Ninjja's nature, so she made one more attempt. "Why don't you let me talk to the head nurse, and then maybe she could talk to the doctor again?"

The nurse gave in to her persistence this time and took her to the head nurse. After a convincing match that lasted about ten minutes, the head nurse went back to her desk and picked up the phone to make the call Ninjja had been waiting for. From a distance, Ninjja couldn't hear any of the conversation, so instead of waiting around, she decided to head back and check on her sister. With a peek into the ward, Ninjja could see that her sister was lying on the bed with her eyes closed. The hope of another day at the hospital had helped her calm down. Ninjja stood still, lest a small movement should disturb the peaceful expression on her face. She glanced back into the corridor and, at the far end, saw Kuru sprinting toward the ward. He was looking visibly excited and seemed like he was all set to sweep his wife off her hospital bed and take her back home on his flying carpet.

Ninjja didn't want to kill his excitement and continued to stand frozen in her place. "Oh, you are still in your hospital robe! Come on!" he exclaimed with some disappointment. Ninjja's sister fluttered her eyelids as she heard this. This emerging interplay of verbal and nonverbal communication was cut short prematurely as the head nurse walked in.

"Sorry, we won't be able to keep the patient any longer than needed. The doctor is not willing to change his view," the head nurse informed them in a definitive tone. It was a big blow to Ninjja's sister's newly acquired comfort. The information was enough to jolt her out of her sleeping position into a visibly agitated state. "Don't you worry; I will give her antianxiety medicine, and she will calm down." The nurse glanced at Ninjja and continued her monologue.

"Giving a medicine for something that could have been solved just through a gradual transition?" Ninjja muttered to herself, annoyed with the turn of events. "How can a health-care system be so mechanical and insensitive?" Ninjja was unable to comprehend the inflexibility that she had just seen. She found herself involuntarily projecting the outcome if the same situation had occurred back home. Despite all the lacunae that had frustrated her in her various encounters with the health-care system in her home country, she was absolutely certain that there would not have been any objection if the patient wanted to spend an extra day at the hospital. The patient's emotional state and overall confidence was something that wouldn't be considered irrelevant (assuming that the patient had the ability to pay for an additional day of hospital stay). *Does this have something to do with the fact that medical expenses are covered by insurance?* A new hypothesis was forming in Ninjja's mind. *Maybe the insurance companies put a lot of pressure on the hospitals to reduce the number of days a patient is required to spend at the hospital. That would directly reduce the cost that the insurance company needs to bear. Considering that the cash has to come from the insurance company, the power that they exercise is potentially substantial.* The rationale for the doctor's decision had started making sense to Ninjja, yet there were several questions that were unanswered. Shouldn't the doctor's judgment be taken as the final call? On the other hand, how would one know that the doctor was not trying to increase the profits for the hospital? Ninjja wondered if the insurance company stipulated norms for the average length of stay under different ailments, and if any deviations required tough explanations that the doctors would much rather avoid than face.

Who drew the line, and where? It did look like there were competing forces at play, which seemed to be companions from a distance. Probably the system hoped that the push and pull due to different incentives would sort themselves out and find a healthy balance. Applying the capitalist philosophy of letting the market forces play themselves out seemed a bit too extreme in a situation where people's lives were involved. There was no way that Ninjja could avoid comparisons between the two health-care models that had now become a part of her experience base. While so far she had been a big admirer of the American health-care system due to its quality and accessibility, the mechanical nature and insensitivity piqued her. The same insurance model that enabled access for the masses and the legal system that helped accountability also created inflexibility as a by-product. The hospital forms replete with legal phrases, the propensity of the nurses and the doctors to offer their opinion in legally correct language, their abstinence from offering any opinion based on judgment, and their reluctance to go beyond the rule book bore testimony to the power that other market partici-pants wielded on the health-care model.

In contrast, the system in India offers a lot more flexibility to the patients who have the means to go to the good hospitals, and the doctors don't seem scared of offering their views based on their best judgment (even with partial and ambiguous information). Ninjja was now musing about the positives of a health-care system that she often derided. She was surprised that she had always taken the posi-tives as a given and the lacunae as a signal of design failure.

Despite the newly identified positives, she knew that this con-fused socialist-elitist model of poor-quality public hospitals and fully independent private hospitals that were affordable to only the privi-leged few was no panacea either. *Is it even possible to design an ideal health-care model?*

"Ninjja, where are you—lost?" She heard Kuru's voice knocking on her head, reminding her of the immediate task at hand. There was no time available to waste. Kuru now no longer bore any signs of the initial excitement he had displayed while entering the ward. Ninjja's sister looked pale with panic, and all the attempts at pacify-ing her were useless. The fear and trauma she expressed were no less than that of a child who was being forcibly taken away from the caring arms of its parents.

The nurse, who probably had a deadline for releasing the pa-tient, was now feeling the pressure. She promptly came back with an antianxiety pill that was going to perform the miracle. Ninjja didn't feel comfortable with this approach and made one last attempt at buying some more time. "I don't think that the medicine will be nec-essary. Let me talk to her alone," she blurted. Fortunately, the nurse obliged and stepped out. Kuru followed the nurse to complete the discharge formalities and to check on his friend, who had bravely of-fered to babysit the infant during this period.

Ninjja had learned about the power of mind over body when her efforts to control her fainting attacks had finally paid off.

She searched her memory from ten years ago.

She had seen several doctors for sudden bouts of breathlessness that would often culminate in fainting. Different doctors prescribed a variety of medicines (including neurological medicines) that did not have any impact. She had discontinued the nerve-calming medi-cation, given the profound drowsiness she experienced. On deeper introspection, she figured that her breathlessness and fainting were triggered by emotional distress. This knowledge was a turning point for her in this battle. The mind finally won and managed to achieve something that no medicine could deliver.

However, at this stage, she was dealing with a weak mind.

She was feeling so helpless with regard to her sister's plight that she couldn't find any words, let alone the words that would do the trick.

Ninjja took a shot in the dark. She hoped that emotional support combined with logic would help her sister get the mental strength needed to avoid additional medication. She controlled the sudden rush of tears and instinctively hugged her sister. There was complete silence for few minutes, and then Ninjja whispered, "Once we are home, you will be able to be with your baby; you will be free!" Ninjja construed the gentle nod and squeeze on her hand as a sign that she had been heard. Building on this small success, Ninjja continued, "You don't need all these monitors. The only critical thing is BP—don't you think?"

There was no response.

"We will buy a BP machine and will keep taking the measurements as many times as we like." Ninjja carried on her monologue while gently patting her sister's head. There was a small pause, and then Ninjja heard an indifferent tone: "OK…but the machines in the market are not reliable." Despite the negative undertone of this response, Ninjja saw this as a hugely positive signal, given the events since the morning. Encouraged, Ninjja continued, "We will buy the best available machine in the market…they should be error-free. And by the way, I also know how to check the pulse…that should help, too."

Even though the last statement was factually incorrect, her confident delivery did help. The dialogue went on for another fifteen minutes, with Ninjja taking up most of the airspace and her sister offering an occasional "Hmm" or a nod. The nurse was back with her full backup plan of antianxiety pills ready to be doled out at the smallest hint of the patient's unwillingness to leave the hospital. To her surprise, she saw the patient in an amicable mood and quickly proceeded to shower praises on Ninjja. "You are a very good sister; how did you manage this? She looks so calm now!" the nurse exclaimed as Kuru was walking in.

His steps were tentative, and his expression looked like that of a child who is greeted with an empty plate after a promise of all his favorite treats.

He was looking down as though afraid of what he might be faced with if he were to change his angle. "Great! Looks like she is all set to go," the nurse chirped again, catching Kuru's attention this time. As Kuru started absorbing the proceedings in the room, the gloom beat a slow retreat from his face.

· · ·

After putting the newly released patient and the attention-seeking infant in their respective comfort zones, Ninjja and Kuru plunged into the sofa and collapsed instantly. After few minutes of nothingness, the events of the day started replaying in Ninjja's subconscious mind. She was glad that she was able to save her sister from at least one extra medication. The power of emotional support for a patient's recovery was not unknown to her; but the fact that it could act as a substitute for medication in some cases was an eye-opener. The new lesson tried to find an empty cell in her memory to deposit itself. The dream sequence had started going into wilder terrain, and she saw herself swimming in the ocean. The waves were getting taller and rougher, and she was almost drowning. The more she tried, the harder it became to breathe. Ninjja suddenly woke up, gasping for breath. She had been asleep for over an hour and a half. Possibly, her physical state was reflecting itself in the dream. "How the hell did I pull through so many days and nights at a stretch?" Ninjja asked herself. As she let go, her worn-out body starting crumbling, and it felt like she would never be able to assemble it to pull herself out of the sofa. Kuru seemed to be in a similar state; the tussle between sleep and consciousness was on!

· · ·

A low-pitched cry had started emanating from one of the bedrooms. The exhausted caregivers, who were still groggy, quietly chose to ignore it. However, the pitch kept increasing one notch higher with every passing minute, and then a loud shriek jolted them out of their stupor and back on their feet.

"Please take her away; quiet her down, please…it is hurting me…I can't stand it." Ninjja's sister was writhing in pain in a half-asleep state. Ninjja scampered to pick up the wailing infant and ran toward the farthest corner of their small apartment to attenuate the noise, while Kuru concentrated on his wife. Now, it was the infant's turn to demonstrate the shift in power. Being ignored for over five minutes was not something that this little one was going to take very kindly to. The rapidly ascending volume was sufficient to scare Ninjja out of her wits and send her bolting out of the main door onto the porch.

Ninjja thought the distance would be enough to insulate her sister from the sound that was causing her so much of discomfort, and she hoped that the neighbors would be kind enough to tolerate this elaborate rendition from her niece. This high-pitched melodrama did settle down after an adequate dosage of cuddling and rocking. Back in the apartment, Ninjja's sister had found some solace after using couple of pillows as ear mufflers and had gone back to sleep.

Once back in the living room, Ninjja and Kuru looked at each other with blank expressions. The feeling of helplessness regarding what lay ahead could not be concealed. The baby could not be programmed to not cry, and there was nothing that they could do to control the hypersensitivity to sound that her sister was suffering from. Having the mother and her baby under the same roof was adding a new dimension to their challenge.

"Let's gear up for phase two of the battle, Kuru," Ninjja uttered unconvincingly as she stepped out to put the baby back in her bassinet.

Ninjja settled back in her sofa with a thud, while Kuru proceeded to make tea to ease their throbbing nerves. The doorbell interrupted them.

• • •

A group of friends who had heard the good news had stopped by to share their best wishes. They were carrying an assortment of bouquets, fruits, and other goodies. The excitement was hard to contain, and it inevitably led to a cacophony of sounds. Their exuberance was silenced by the screaming protest from her sister. The pleas to "shut up" got a bit embarrassing for the hosts and shocked the cheerful visitors. Kuru gulped down his tea before proceeding to offer an explanation, while Ninjja hurried inside to calm down her sister. Fortunately, the baby was in a benign mood and chose not to add its own symphony to the ensuing confusion.

Five

The Reality Check

The house felt like a continuous factory where the operations halted only when Ninjja slumped on the bed beside her sister and Kuru fell asleep on the rocking chair while trying to put the baby to sleep.

· · ·

It was time to administer the first morning dosage of medicine to Ninjja's sister. The new blood-pressure machine was still a novelty, even though Kuru had diligently used it three times already. He arranged all his assortments from the medical kit on the table and proceeded to attach the digital device on her sister's arm. Despite several trials, the device was showing a strange behavior—it didn't show any reading. To be doubly sure, Kuru tried it few more times and either got no reading or got an error message. Given the track record of digital BP monitors, he wrote this one off as another bad buy. "Something has gone wrong with this one; you should take all your medicines in any case," he said to Ninjja's sister. She obediently started popping the pills one by one. As she picked up the BP medicine, Kuru instinctively stopped her. "Wait a minute. Let me check if this machine works on me."

The BP machine offered a reading that sounded reasonable. That did merit some attention. "Ninjja, let me check your BP." Ninjja extended her left arm, and voilà, the BP measurement popped up.

"Looks like it is working again." Kuru got excited and tried it again on his wife. The results didn't change—there wasn't any reading.

"This feels a bit odd," Ninjja remarked. "What should we do about the BP medicine? The nurse said that we need to be extra particular about this medicine to keep the blood pressure under control. Maybe we should just go ahead."

"Yes, I guess," Kuru concurred tentatively.

"What if we wait till we get another instrument? It won't take more than half an hour, right?" Ninjja suggested. Kuru immediately sprang into action as though he had been waiting for a way out. He was back within twenty-five minutes with a supposedly better version of the instrument. However, there seemed to be some discord between the instruments and her sister. The same story repeated itself. Two data points were enough to ring an alarm bell, and Kuru remarked, "I think we should wait. In any case, we have an appointment with her GP in couple of hours. Why not check with her?" Ninjja was worried about the blood pressure shooting up, yet her instinct told her that Kuru was probably making the right call.

• • •

The BP medicine was looming large in the background while Kuru and Ninjja's sister went out to meet the GP. The time was moving rather slowly. Like every other wait, this one ended when Ninjja received a call from Kuru.

"Thank God we didn't give her the BP medicine!" he squeaked triumphantly and paused.

Ninjja's anxiety and curiosity forced her to react. "No puzzles, please! What happened?"

"Actually, her blood pressure had become so low—eighty over fifty-five (80/55)—that it was below the accuracy range of the digital BP machine. If we had given her the medicine for high BP as advised at the hospital, she may have collapsed!"

"Now what?" Ninjja blurted out, unsure of whether the situation was under control or if it required another round of serious attention.

"We need to give her lots of saline water and monitor her blood pressure closely. If things get worse, we may need to hospitalize her." The reply came almost instantly. Ninjja was amazed with the poise that Kuru demonstrated at this moment. The message that she was hearing and the calm tone of Kuru's voice did not seem to match up.

Perhaps the recent victory of Kuru's instinct-driven decision was supporting his nerves. As the gravity of the situation sank in, she found it difficult to control her emotional reaction. "This looks bizarre! A warning at the hospital to expect huge fluctuations in BP would have been good!" Ninjja responded in a critical tone. She continued her reprimand as though she were speaking to the curt nurse and not to Kuru.

"I can't believe it; I actually asked about this and was told not to bother about monitoring. The high-BP medicine had to be adminstered as prescribed. This is the height of callousness. This is murderous!"

Ninjja was now fuming and had mentally strangled the overconfident nurse for the hundredth time when Kuru interjected, "Ninjja, cool down. We can't change the past. Please start preparing a large bottle of lemon water with loads of sugar and salt. I will pick up a manual BP instrument as well on the way." This forward-looking, positive speech helped Ninjja to get to a simmering stage. Her attention was diverted by the baby's thunderous cry, and Ninjja's bout of anger met a premature death.

•   •   •

Kuru and Ninjja got busy with demystifying the manual blood-pressure machine and were pleased to find that it wasn't difficult to use after all. The calibration with their own blood pressures gave them the confidence to try it on the patient.

They were jubilant to detect similar readings as the doctor's recent findings, though the reading per se didn't merit any celebration. Without much delay, the combo of rest and fresh lime along with hourly monitoring was unleashed. Signs of positive movement started showing up in the evening, making the potential ominous hospital visit feel like a passing bad dream.

•   •   •

The operations of the day petered out by nine in the evening.

For the first time in over two weeks, Ninjja got the opportunity to think about other people around her. She thought of calling her parents, who were still blissfully unaware of the actual situation. Periodic phone calls with occasional laughter and the baby's wailing in the background had been enough to convince them that it was "life as usual" on the other side of the Pacific.

Ninjja was surprised as well as happy with their naïveté and had no intention of breaking the pretense till she got back home. After the usual "Yeah, all is well…everyone else is sleeping…" Ninjja learned that her mother's fracture was healing well, and she might be able to travel in another two weeks. Spurred on with the good news, Ninjja felt that she could enhance her circle of activity and remembered that she had brought a laptop. After the usual struggle with the multicountry adapter, her laptop got the required juice to be able to come back to life.

A few minutes in front of that blank screen reminded her of the feeling of nothingness that had been all-encompassing since that fateful call from Kuru.

Despite being an IT professional, Kuru was not into establishing elaborate security systems for his wireless network, enabling Ninjja to easily get connected with the virtual world.

In an agenda-free surfing mode, she robotically went to her office network and clicked on e-mail. Suddenly, a never-ending string of "ding-ding-ding" pierced through her eardrums, forcing her out of her newly attained semblance of peace. "What the…" Ninjja grumbled as she struggled to find the volume-control key on her laptop.

Her e-mail was set up to give an alarm for the arrival of each new e-mail, and now, with over four hundred e-mails finding their way in, the mild alarm had morphed itself into unstoppable, loud temple bells. Ninjja was still running for cover when her attention was caught by Arv's name popping up few times in the inbox. She remembered that she was supposed to meet Arv ten days earlier and had completely forgotten about it in this pandemonium.

She was overcome by a sense of guilt. She knew that she would be able to read or send any of the e-mails only when tons of megabytes of attachments were comfortably at home on her laptop. That could easily take the whole night. Ninjja felt that the voice route would be in order to recover the situation.

. . .

Arv answered after just one ring and was curious to know who was calling from an unknown international number. "Oh, OK, so it is you! I am glad to know that you are still alive," he responded coldly. Ninjja's apologies were cut short abruptly as Arv went on, "I am sure you have a solid excuse yet again. Your phone was unreachable… your office receptionist had no clue…I have been worried sick, but who cares?" Arv thundered, and he disconnected the call.

She tried again, but there was no response. After the fourth try, Arv gave in and picked up the phone.

"My sister had a brain hemorrhage," Ninjja bursted out.
The sharp statement indeed had a piercing impact. She could feel Arv's shock on the other end of the phone connection as his voice transformed into that of complete compassion.

"Did you say brain hemorrhage?" he repeated slowly, as though trying to absorb what he had just heard. Ninjja packed the events of over two weeks into the next fifteen minutes and left Arv gasping for breath. The reconciliatory note was clear as they bid good-bye to each other. While Arv had forgiven her, Ninjja was still disappointed with her own behavior. "I did inform my team at work about an emergency. I did reach out to Uma to help out my parents. Why didn't I think of informing Arv?" Ninjja asked herself. "Possibly in a crisis, one can remember just the immediate commitments." This was the only weak reason that she could conjecture to rationalize her actions.

The clock had struck eleven, and the much-awaited sleep was nowhere in sight. Ninjja thought of doing one more check on her sister's blood pressure and pulled out the instrument from the medicine cupboard. The new reading (110/70) reaffirmed her comfort. With the baby sleeping soundly and showing absolutely no indications of any impending demands, Ninjja was reassured that she was redundant, at least for the time being.

• • •

The sudden lull felt very strange. Once one gets something that one has been craving, one doesn't know what to do with it. Ninjja was in a similar situation. The sudden peace was getting difficult to handle. She parked herself on the plush reclining chair and closed her eyes.

Her mind started running through the many twists and turns of the past few weeks and paused at every corner to carefully disentangle itself. Once she had stepped back, she could see the darkness and light coexisting all through the tunnel that had completely escaped her when she was in the middle of it. The irony was that although she was thankful to the medical fraternity for saving her sister's life, that same medical fraternity had potentially created the situation in the first place by ignoring the early warning signals (the OB/GYN had chosen to ignore the 170/85 BP coupled with headaches just a day before the incident as a normal postdelivery complication!). Ninjja thought about the several actions that they had taken along the way, either through instinct or through reasoning, which saved them from potentially catastrophic consequences.

Was there some method to this madness? Was it possible to distill some learning from the ordeal that could help her or others in the future?

She was too comfortable in her position to leave the reclining chair, so she stretched her hand instead to grab the laptop bag. It required some sustained stretching and ingeniousness to use the nearby pen to pull the bag's handle. Ninjja reached out for her yellow diary, which always reclaimed its spot in her bag.

She glanced through some of the earlier thoughts that she had jotted down and felt that she had used some of those lessons automatically in this situation as well, such as asking questions when one was unsure, not assuming that nurses were always right, and being vigilant toward any anomalies.

A potential narcotics addiction could not have been avoided if Ninjja had been just a receiver of instructions from the attending medical staff. Yet there were several first-time bone-chilling experiences that she wished she had never encountered. Ninjja was fortunate enough to be able to come out unscathed and was at liberty of adding to her learning repository. "I am so archaic...at some point I should convert my yellow diary to an electronic file," Ninjja muttered as she reunited her multipurpose pen with the famous yellow diary to start writing. She had no idea how prolific she was until her ninth point gave way to several others.

—◊—

My Survival Mantra

1. Don't assume that your regular physician will always know what is right for you.
2. When in doubt, seek a second opinion.
3. Always have health insurance and carefully select the plan.
4. Don't rush to a specialist based on your perceived issue.
5. Overseas insurance is not a blank check.
6. A balanced lifestyle holds the secret of many a cure.
7. In situations of emergency (e.g., an accident), don't run to the closest hospital.
8. Several diseases may have stress as the underlying cause.
9. **Watch out for medicine addiction!** Unfortunately, one can become addicted to lifesaving or pain-management drugs without actively engaging in drug abuse. For example, drugs used in cases of acute pain at times have narcotics as an important ingredient, which can cause addiction. These medicines may be unavoidable evils in some situations, while in others they may

be doled out to the overanxious or to the perceived zero-tolerance patients as an insurance policy against frustrating follow-up calls or consultations. What can we do? In either situation, read about the ingredients, reconfirm if a milder alternative could work, and watch out for any symptoms of addiction, such as cravings for the medicine, trance, or odd behavior, and alert your doctor. Even in situations where such drugs are indispensable, doctors can manage the risk of addiction by changing or alternating medicines, provided one is alert enough to raise the alarm when needed.

10. Emotional support as a substitute to some medicines? In several situations, neither the patients nor the doctors have the patience to invest the time needed to manage with minimum medication, especially when the problems are psychosomatic. There are enough drugs available for a quick turn-around so that the patient is happily back to the "normal course," while the healthcare provider gets maximum returns for the time invested. How about the long-term effects of this approach on the CNS (central nervous system)? If a frenzied anxiety attack could be managed without the anti-anxiety pills, there must be enough situations where adequate emotional support could lead to a much more stable and sustainable

recovery. It is time to step back if you or someone close to you is taking medication for anxiety, depression, phobias, or any other psychosomatic problems. The power of family support and strength should not be underestimated. This is not to say that all the medication should be stopped, but the need for a discussion with the doctor on behavioral aspects can't be ruled out. It does take a lot of mental strength and energy to intervene in such a situation, and every family may not have a "rock" to lean on. Seeking help from a therapist or counselor on how to best manage the situation can complement the treatment for speed as well as for sustainability of recovery. The final decision is yours, but stepping back and thinking about the right course of action should not be optional.

II. Don't take medicines in blind faith. There is no escape from having your antennae up when you or someone close to you is undergoing treatment. The degree of monitoring depends on the severity of the disease or ailment and the patient's current status (e.g., unstable versus steady state). Clearly severe ailments that are just triggered would require the most careful monitoring for administering the medicines. As an example, while a regular dosage of a blood-pressure medicine might be normal for a person who is in a steady state of hypertension, it may not be right if the high blood pressure is a new phenomenon (it could be due to some other ailment, such as anxiety). In such a situation, it has to be watched carefully before blindly taking the medicine. The hospital environment versus the home environment also makes a difference. One needs to watch out for any adverse effects or faster changes than expected and adjust the dosage in consultation with the doctor.

At this point, Ninjja was struggling hard to keep her management-consulting hat away so that she didn't end up drawing a two-by-two matrix! Finally, she had to give in. The words were taking too long to express what she had to say, and despite the verbiage, they were not lucid. She started wondering if being linguistically challenged was a key criterion for becoming a management consultant.

However, the bullet points and pictorial language that the consultants have invented seems to get through to the clients much more easily, Ninjja rationalized, and she proceeded to complete her thought process.

My Survival Mantra

Maybe the attached chart could help in deciding the extent and nature of intervention needed:

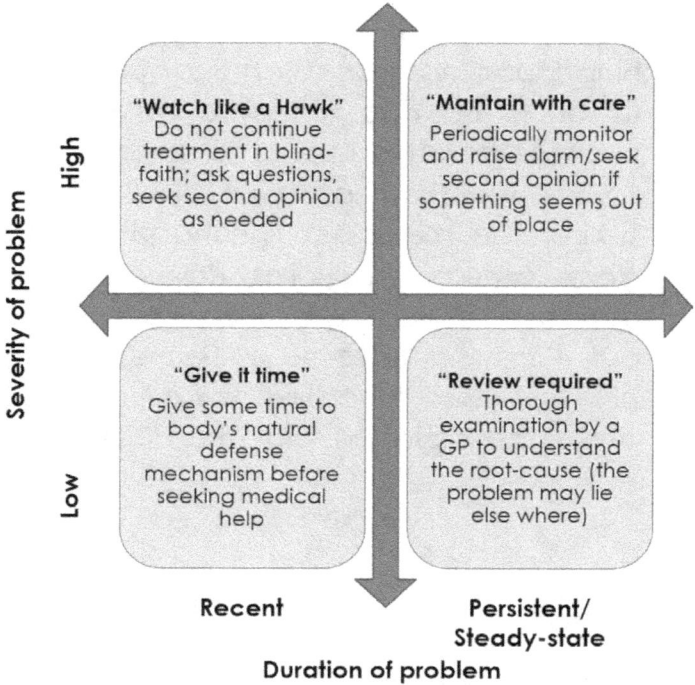

Framework to decide the level of attention

12. **There is no utopian health-care system that exists.** The belief that if we were receiving treatment in the developed world, every-thing would have been perfect, is a myth. It is easy to blame the health-care sys-tem and externalize the issue if things don't work out the way they are expected to. Like everything else in life, there are pros and cons to every model, and the extent may vary. Depending on the context, one may find oneself at the deep end of the pool even in a better-perceived health-care system. This is not to say that no attempts

should be made to improve the health-care system (especially in the developing world), but while one is on the receiving end, neither blind faith nor utter contempt helps.

In countries with multitiered health-care systems, one may have the option of choosing; elsewhere it might come as given. There are trade-offs on multiple dimensions (e.g., affordability, access, flexibility, and accountability). The key is to be aware of the trade-offs that one is likely to face with one's choice of health-care model. Once one is aware, one's expectations and the nature of one's actions can be tailored accordingly.

For example, if one is getting treated in a system with very clear processes that is heavily driven by market mechanisms (e.g., the United States), though the quality of care may be reasonably good, it is unlikely that the doctors and nurses will step out of their boundary conditions to accommodate the patient's unique situation or special requests. Perhaps the fear of lawsuits and pressure from insurance agencies constrain them. While it does force tremendous accountability, it also drives them to risk-averse behavior. In such a scenario one should be mentally prepared for multitudes of tests before the diagnosis. Also, one needs to be careful about overmedication and ask about the purpose of each medicine in the prescription. In some cases, additional medication for short-term anxiety, sleep disorders, or pain may not be needed, but it might be pre-scribed for a quicker turnaround. In some cases, you might be released from the hospital sooner than warranted. (The doctors might find it hard to fit your bill in the predefined expense norms, or the process metrics compel them to do so.) Be mentally prepared for this. An assumption that "released from the hospital = doing fine" can be lethal. Be sure to ensure close monitoring of vitals and any odd symptoms. Call the doctor if something doesn't seem right. Erring on the side of being overcautious can never hurt!

Don't forget that if one is unable to afford an insurance policy, filing for bankruptcy due to a medical exigency may not be too farfetched.

If one is glad to be in a system that offers universal access at affordable costs, one has to be prepared for long waiting times and less at-tention from the attending doctor.

Then, there is a pseudomarket-driven model, where there are a range of options, depending on what you can afford (e.g., India). At one end are premium/superspecialty branded chains, and at the other are the government-funded hospitals. If the market mechanism doesn't push for strong ac-countability despite autonomy, an assumption that "higher price = higher quality" can be detrimental. Without pressure from insurance companies and with no fear of a regulator or legal liabilities, one's well-being would be mostly a function of the hospital's goodwill and one's luck. One can draw solace from the fact that in the premium hospitals, the quality of doctors and the medical devises is likely to be best in class. One important thing to understand is that doctors are not the only people who make a difference to one's treatment. Often, doctors don't even have control over the nurses and attendants, who are the final touch point in final care. They have a different, parallel hierarchy.

A lesser-known fact is that a large chunk of medical errors happen due to negligence in simple things, like sanitation standards, administering wrong medications, and lack of communication between the doctors and nursing staff. These can be corrected only through higher accountability. The importance of being extra careful toward some of these basics and asking questions or raising an alarm could not be further underscored, especially in a situation when the patient is admitted to the hospital. The good news is that the likelihood of the hospital staff being receptive and responsive to questions is going to be much higher for a customer who is paying their price. Also, the doctors may be willing to offer their opinions based on best judgment (even with partial data) if you ask.

On the other end of the spectrum is the state-managed model. It is easy to write volumes on the pathetic state of government-funded public hospitals in the developing countries, but the fact is that they are still serving millions of patients who can't even afford daily meals. As an example, if we view the contribution of over thirty-five thousand government hospitals and clinics in India, it is not a small feat. They treated over eleven million cases of acute diarrheal diseases, over twenty-five million cases of acute respiratory infection, over one point five million cases of malaria, and so on at minimal costs, according to the Ministry of Health and Family Welfare. The need for removing graft, better review mechanisms, incentive systems, and performance-driven financial aid can't be wished away, but only after giving due recognition to the public servants who operate in extremely tough conditions with meager salaries.

It is unlikely that anyone who is reading this will go to a government hospital by choice; but if a necessity (e.g., an accident), forces this upon you, don't panic! The doctors who are operating with scarce resources on a daily basis have a rich experience for emergency responses. Needless to say, a follow-up at a better-equipped hospital will be important.

See Figure 1 in the Appendix for a pictorial representation of the key dimensions of trade-offs.

—m—

. . .

The clock had struck 1:00 a.m., and Ninjja's faculties were slowing down. She was sad that the experience that she described above would more often than not come at a huge emotional and financial cost to the recipient. She was glad with her attempt, yet there was something that was bothering her. All her lessons were going to only help people who had the ability to pay. She was feeling blanked out in terms of actions that the financially challenged could take to utilize the health-care systems available to their best advantage. She closed her eyes, hoping to get a deep insight in her dreams...

. . .

Ninjja felt a sudden chill in the air. As she bundled up for warmth, a clinking sound brought her back to her senses. The collection of motley things, like her diary, her pen, and the purse with its further assortment of things rarely used, had all tumbled down to the floor when she turned. It was four o'clock. Ninjja realized that she had been sleeping in the reclining chair with all this stuff on her lap. In a dazed state, she tried to pick up items scattered on the floor and reached out for the blanket thrown on the sofa.

Ninjja had barely resumed her nap when the infant decided to change the definition of morning silence.

. . .

Unfortunately, Ninjja's tired brain couldn't conjure up any insights on the problem that she had gone to sleep with; instead, she found her brain pondering the conversation with Arv. His anger, his concern, and his understanding had touched her somewhere and offered an inexplicable emotional comfort. It did bring a smile to her face.

* * *

Strong sunlight was piercing the open curtains. Ninjja slowly woke up with a happy feeling. The morning cup of tea brought her lost alertness back, and with it also came the bite of reality. Ninjja was now admonishing herself for a momentary lapse of consciousness (even though it was in a dream) and for letting feelings creep over her mind. *Am I brain-dead, or what? How can I even imagine in my wildest dreams that Arv actually cares about me? Mr. Casanova is probably busy with a dinner date at this very moment with someone from his renewable stock of girlfriends! In all likelihood he will call me in a month for love advice when things are not going his way.* She almost slapped herself.

The daily operations had begun in full force, and the energy needed in cajoling her sister for breakfast, drinking milk, and taking her regular dosage of medicines helped Ninjja completely disentangle from the slipup that her brain had committed accidentally. The day offered a joyous moment when her sister expressed a desire to go out in the park for a stroll. She still had headaches, but she didn't look terrified at the thought of getting exposed to noise while venturing out in a public place. She also occasionally cuddled the baby and expressed her sadness and helplessness for not being able to feed the baby—all good indicators of normal behavior.

* * *

Later that evening, Kuru announced, "Guess what! From tomorrow, we are going to have someone else in the house as well. We have got a daytime *nanny* cum *cook!*"

With this news, the excitement level in the room was equivalent to that of someone who sees a ship on the horizon after being marooned on an island for years.

Ninjja's imagination had already started flying toward innumerable things that she could do with the time that would be freed up. A celebration tea was made, and the calorie count of cheese-stuffed, fried jalapeños was conveniently ignored for the moment. While nothing had actually changed that evening in terms of the effort required to keep things under control, Ninjja was feeling much lighter mentally. She found herself picking up the TV remote for the first time in the past three weeks and thinking about which program to watch, rather than being on guard for the slightest disturbance that might signal trouble. Later that night, Ninjja's "talkative form" was in full action as she called up her parents, her friends, Arv, Uma, Rohan…the list was fairly long! After becoming exhausted with the spurt of activity to celebrate the imminent breathing space, Ninjja fell asleep.

The next day delivered well on the expected respite.

Ninjja's thoughts went back to the unfinished agenda from two days ago: *What could the financially challenged do to use the available health-care model to their best advantage?* It was obvious that they would need to optimize under a much higher number of constraints like fewer options, lack of awareness, inability to fix the root causes of malnutrition, hygiene, and financial burden of related travel and accommodation expenses and so on. The service providers like doctors, hospitals, nurses, insurance companies, pharma companies all needed to make money, as most people and enterprises do.

The puzzle seemed to be getting more complex for Ninjja. *Am I being devoid of all realism when I am thinking of providing medical attention to people who don't even get food to eat?* Ninjja wondered. In a flash, she was reminded of all the idealistic articles and research papers that preached the "moral code of conduct" for governments and institutions. She shuddered at the thought of even remotely falling in the category of "Thou shall do this…" pedestal-riding authors…and then she wrote down her most critical question:

WHAT IS THE VALUE AT STAKE?

Beyond humanitarian grounds, is there any other value to the stakeholders like governments, global welfare organizations, for-profit players, and so on if the health of these poor individuals were to improve? She was looking for another platform to broaden the appeal to the stakeholders and hopefully find a win-win solution.

Having a healthier workforce should mean more productivity, which should equal more value for the nation and the individual, her logical mind argued. The thought piqued her curiosity, and she resorted to googling to see if there were any others who had similar brainwaves. She came across couple of interesting articles on the topic. One had an American perspective and claimed that a comparison of wealth between two sets of individuals with differing health (all other parameters being equal) could be as much as three times, or the equivalent of *about $450,000 over the lifetime.* The other one was more academic and had concocted elaborate equations to prove that increasing the health quotient of a nation should contribute to an increase in wealth overall. Though there was no quantification, Ninjja felt some comfort that her thought process was not completely bizarre.

Encouraged by her findings, she felt that at least at the system level, it should be possible to cover these costs through the tangible and intangible benefits of a healthier workforce. She picked a simple example of a poor worker who forms the backbone of any Indian household—the cleaning maid.

The laborious work, coupled with poor living standards, often meant that such people had a much lower productive life (shorter by ten to fifteen years) compared to their healthier counterparts. That would translate to $10,000 to $20,000 in lost earnings of the poor maid over a lifetime without even accounting for inflation. The financial effect would be further magnified as the maid in question would not be in a position to send her children for higher education or upgrade their skills and increase their contribution to the economy or to themselves. Going by the government's statistics of 30 percent of people being qualified as poor, even if we consider one working person per household, it translates to sixty million individuals or more. Applying the $10,000 rule, the numbers quickly multiply to $600 billion or more over a decade. If anything, Ninjja felt that this was a very conservative estimate, as this ignored many of the multiplicative aspects, such as the following:

- Enhancing GDP as people moved to higher value-added jobs.
- Growth due to addressing the labor shortage: In a situation where every urban household was complaining about shortage of domestic help, where the construction industry was blaming the project delays on labor shortage, where every industry was struggling to find enough semiskilled and skilled workmen, and wage inflation was rife, increase in productive

life would definitely add to the competitiveness of the industry and increase GDP growth.
- Above all, there was a nonmonetary aspect of people being able to live a better life that was priceless.

Ninjja rested her case. She felt comfortable that there was enough value on the table that all the stakeholders could benefit from, and she felt that the job of precise assessment of value of all of the above benefits should be best left to the better offices of economists.

Now came the most difficult part: the *how*. She was now moving down from the realm of strategy to the tougher domain of reality. Creating a win-win for all the stakeholders to achieve the goal of *minimum sufficiency* within constraints was not going to be easy.

Was the available funding sufficient? As with any heavy and difficult topic, her brain had started freezing.

Maybe I need to relax a bit to get some more fresh ideas, she tried to console herself. Instinctively, she found herself dialing Arv's number. "Hi, who is calling?" she heard his usual chirpy voice.

"Hope I am not disturbing you." Ninjja tried to be polite.

"Actually, you are," Arv quipped. "I have just reached the office, and there are twenty urgent e-mails waiting for me. But I am sure the e-mails can be comfortable in the inbox for some more time, having spent the whole night here," he continued in the same breath, without giving Ninjja any time to apologize for her bad timing.

"How are things over there? When will you be back?" Arv provided her with the comfortable path to start the conversation.

After the pleasantries, the latest status updates, and highlights of Arv's tumultuous dating life, Ninjja moved over to the topic that had been bothering her.

"How do we expect the developing countries to pay for the health-care of their poor people? Where will the funds come from? Even if they spend the same percentage of their GDP as developed nations, the quantum per person would be so small that it can be easily forgotten. What do you think, Arv?"

"Whoa…hold on! I don't think I am ready for such a heavy topic right in the morning." Arv was surprised. However, he soon regained his wit and added, "I have no idea what the answer should be…but here are my two cents. It is not just about how much you spend, but how you spend it."

Was this one of Arv's usual casual one-liners, or was there a deeper meaning to it? Ninjja was confused. For a change, she decided to be "thoughtful" about the twenty urgent e-mails waiting in Arv's inbox and chose to ignore her instinct to pick up an immediate argument with him.

As she put the phone down, the deep-sounding one-liner was still ringing in her head. She vaguely remembered reading about a comparison between Japan and the United States in the health-care context that showed that Japan was able to achieve more with less. To satisfy the curiosity of her numerical brain, she looked for statistics. She found that Japan spent less than half of what the United States spent per capita on health and yet had a much higher average life expectancy.

Spending more on health care did not necessarily translate to better health. Ninjja was not surprised to see diminishing returns on increased spending. She had seen this happen across several industries and companies.

Similarly, China's spending on health care in terms of percentage of GDP was comparable to several other middle-income countries, but the results were dramatically different—better life expectancy and lower infant mortality to name a few. So what was working in these places?

Was the difference due to better government controls or fundamentally different health-care models, or was there something else, such as the cultural fact that Asians don't run for a medicine at the first signal and allow nature to do some work?

Alas, she couldn't find any reliable "health-care spending efficiency and effectiveness" metrics that could be dissected to draw out the best practices.

However, one thing was clear: spending more alone couldn't be the answer.

· · ·

As she continued her exploration, she stumbled upon a striking piece of information: "leakage." One of the articles mentioned, "In the developed world 10–25 percent of funds for procurement get lost due to leakages and in developing countries, up to 89 percent leakage of procurement and operational costs had been observed."

This was a stunning revelation. This seemed worse than the electricity theft in India that was estimated at 25 to 40 percent! *Given this magnitude, shouldn't all the renowned global agencies be directing their advice to plug the leakages rather than berating the governments to allocate more funds toward health care?* Ninjja was perplexed. As she read more, she found enough articles, theoretical analysis, and recommendations by reputed agencies like the WHO, the World Bank, IMF, and academicians to address this issue. *It is clear that the efforts are being made, but can one expect to fill a bucket by increasing the tap opening, when the bucket has a missing bottom (and not a small pinhole leak)?* The magnitude of the challenge had shaken her. She didn't get the feeling that the initiatives and efforts were in line with the gravity of the situation. The news media seemed quiet in most countries. A few sporadic news articles in a SEA country talked about a 70 percent loss of government funds and lamented on the "shortfall of medicines" in government-run centers, overcharging up to 100 percent for the drugs, and "spurious medicines" that left the health-care staff to struggle on the ground without ammunition.

Ninjja was crestfallen! Did that mean that the situation was beyond salvation till the core issue of corruption was fixed? She felt the desperation of a person lost in an Alaskan forest, who, after walking for the whole day in subzero temperatures, found himself back in the same spot where he started. (Remember the movie *The Edge*, starring Antony Hopkins?)

Ninjja was vigorously tapping the pen on her head when she heard the infant rumbling for attention.

· · ·

The cry continued to build up, as the nanny had chosen to ignore the baby till she could finish the work at hand.

"The baby should be your first priority; everything else is secondary," Ninjja rebuked the half-receptive nanny as she picked up the infant, who desperately needed a diaper change. After completing the uninspiring task of changing the soiled diaper, Ninjja got an unexpected reward: a lovely smile from the tiny form. It made her day!

• • •

The nanny, who was more interested in housekeeping and cooking than in being a nanny, announced that lunch was ready. Ninjja couldn't remember the last time that she had actually eaten a proper meal on the dining table. Despite the deviations from the expected model of home support, the outcome on the food dimension was positively surprising. "I can live with the diaper changes and making formula in exchange for the good food and vacuum-cleaned apartment!" Ninjja murmured to Kuru as they sat down for lunch. Ninjja's sister had become extremely moody and chose to eat in her bed instead. Her habit of snapping even without slightest provocation had begun to worry Ninjja and Kuru.

"Tomorrow is an important day, and we should hope to get an all-clear signal from the doctor after the MRI. I will also discuss this mood-swing issue with the doctor. I am sure this is a temporary phenomenon," Kuru said.

"Hmm...then I will also need to make a call on my return plans. I am supposed to fly off in two days," Ninjja replied, trying to remember the date-change rules of her airline.

• • •

Ninjja was back in her thinking chair. However depressing the situation might sound, the fact that having a healthier population was in the interest of governments and was the dream of every person living on this planet offered her a ray of hope. There had to be some way of controlling the leakage and improving efficiencies!

She started thinking about the models that government had followed in other strategic industries where a stand-alone investment by a private player was unviable due to the socioeconomic constraints. The models were still evolving, but at least they provided enough evidence that instilling the principles of a "market mechanism" enabled better efficiencies and provided a path for faster investment growth.

Thinking of the grim power-sector example in India, Ninjja remembered the time when government backing of a "cost recovery" formula with fixed returns (since the end-user price was capped) allowed several power plants to come up. However, the "cost recovery" inherently meant that companies were not incentivized to worry about the efficiency. This led to abuse of the provision by several participants that compelled the government to introduce minimum utilization and fuel-efficiency norms. Significant change in output parameters was observed since then, proving the point that governments might be better off creating the enabling conditions and policies rather than trying to run operations themselves.

Ninjja tried to come up with a probable reason for the observed leakages:

Inability to attract the best talent combined with inadequate rewards and punishments for performance in an almost guaranteed job unfortunately created ample incentives for abuse of power at the system level.

Is it even possible to recover from this degradation? she wondered. She was staring at two dramatically different options: rebuild or reinforce. Her civil-engineer friend had told her once that at times, it is easier and safer to construct a new building rather than adding reinforcements to a crumbling tower.

The key question to think about was, *How crumbly is the tower?*

Ninjja was now talking aloud and wished that she had the ear of the policy makers.

She felt it was time that governments and global agencies did a critical assessment of the health and salvage potential of the existing publicly funded health-care systems and took a call on reinforce versus rebuild.

Before sinking in further resources and throwing more good money after bad, there should be clarity on relative emphasis: cleaning up the existing system versus constructing and experimenting with newer models of public-private partnerships for higher efficacy and faster reach to the needy.

The doorbell interrupted her.

It brought in a most welcome visitor: the housekeeper. Ninjja had mentally struck off "nanny" as a descriptor for this authoritarian lady to save herself from the trouble of expectation mismatch. The morning cup of tea was all that she wanted at this time. Since the time she had embarked upon the issue of health-care for the underprivileged, it was getting increasingly difficult to find solutions in isolation.

Ninjja knew that, often, attempts to find the perfect solution for complex issues obstructed implementation of a good enough solution that could have made a substantial difference. She wanted to avoid this trap.

She recalled a famous quote by Confucius—"Life is really simple, but we insist on making it complicated"—to find direction.

Suddenly, despite the blur, she could see actions that different stakeholders could take, independently or collectively, to make a difference. Ninjja strongly believed that the sum of proposed independent actions would definitely be more than no action at all and would augment the collective action, if that were ever to take off.

• • •

She was interrupted by Kuru's agitated voice. He seemed upset with something. "Why aren't you listening? We need to go for your routine checkup, and we will be late if you don't get up now." Ninjja popped in to find that her sister was sitting there with an expressionless face, refusing to even acknowledge what Kuru had been requesting, let alone act on it. Ignoring the oddity of her conduct, Ninjja set about tackling the immediate task: cajoling her sister to concede. The task of thinking about actions by different groups was curtailed even before it had begun!

• • •

After the two of them had left, Ninjja felt a desperate need to get fresh air. The only option was to hope that the housekeeper's human instincts would supersede her sternness should the baby demand any immediate attention. As a token insurance, Ninjja chose to walk within hearing distance to not miss any loud wailing.

Ninjja tried hard to refocus her energy on the topic on hand, but the events of the morning were causing her discomfort. *Is this some sort of relapse?* She was scared to even harbor such a thought. Her readings on the Internet did not make her any wiser. Three hours had gone by when she heard Kuru's voice again at the door.

He walked in, complaining, "Ninjja, please figure out what she wants. I don't know what she is upset about. The nurses got tired of waiting for her at the MRI room...she hasn't been talking to me, either."

"What did the doctor say?" Ninjja asked to deflect the issue.

"The doctor says she is doing fine; he reviewed the MRI report and said there is no reason to worry," Kuru replied in a flat tone.

At the risk of irritating Kuru further, Ninjja continued, "What did he have to say about her odd conduct?"

"What can the doctor do about it if she is upset with something and doesn't want to talk about it? In any case, the doctor did talk to her and didn't mention that anything was wrong," Kuru retorted.

Ninjja didn't think it was the right time to press the matter further and chose to change the topic to something more pleasant. "The baby behaved very well today. She played with me and didn't cry even a bit. Look at her." She handed the baby over to her sister. Ninjja glanced at her sister, who did not look too well. Her face bore the expression of a drug addict who was on a high. She stared at the baby blankly and did not react when the baby smiled. The analogy of the drug addict made Ninjja's heart stop for a second, and a thought struck her in a flash. *Are all the medicines that she is taking messing her up?*

While Ninjja was eager to uncover what was going on with her sister, she knew that prodding too quickly could be risky. She asked her sister to rest. While pulling the comforter over her, Ninjja gently asked, "Do you have a headache? Should I give you a head massage?"

After couple of minutes of silence, Ninjja got her reply. "No, I don't know what is happening. Feels like my head is spinning. I didn't want to go to the hospital. The MRI room looked so far off…I was afraid that I would fall. Everyone wanted me to hurry things up…" Her sister was speaking very slowly.

"Then why didn't you ask for Kuru's help?"

Again there was a long pause. "He is upset with me for some reason. So I didn't feel like bothering him further."

"I thought you had gone off to sleep when you didn't answer my question," Ninjja continued, hoping to find answers for the long, scary pauses.

"I have to think before talking," came the slow reply, the pause being even longer than the previous ones.

"Hmm…OK, you need to sleep to get back your energy," Ninjja said unconvincingly and closed the blinds. She sat near the top corner of the bed and put a hand on her sister's head. Ninjja wasn't sure if she was doing this to offer some comfort to her sister or if she was actually hoping to calm her own agitated nerves.

Ninjja was glued to her position with no sense of the clock ticking by. The housekeeper announced that lunch was served and pulled her out from the whirlwind of scary thoughts. Ninjja didn't feel like waking her sister up from the deep, peaceful sleep that she seemed to be in.

At the lunch table, she picked up the discussion with Kuru again. "Looks like her brain is taking much longer to process things. That is why she doesn't respond to our questions quickly enough. Also, she is dizzy and doesn't feel in control when she is walking…" Ninjja paused to take a sip of water.

Kuru's expression now bore concern instead of irritation as he put his spoon back on the plate.

"I think she has also become supersensitive, and when she feels that we are losing patience or are getting irritated with her, she just goes back into a shell to shut us out," Ninjja continued.

"I don't understand this. How could the doctor say that she is doing fine, in that case?" Kuru was confused and worried. "I am not even sure if we can speak to him again and discuss this till we get the next appointment."

"I wonder if this is the impact of the steroids that she is taking," said Ninjja. "I don't know much about this, but I have heard that these medicines can do strange things to your body. I was given some steroids for a short while to treat an allergy, and I must say, I didn't feel perfectly normal during that period."

The unknown is always scarier than the "known devil." Though the situation hadn't changed even one bit, Kuru felt a bit relaxed, as there was a potential reason that they could attach to the unknown. After gulping down his lunch quickly, he went to the phone again to try for the doctor. The nurse at the other end took down the request and mentioned that she would try to get a hold of the doctor once he was free. She had conveniently refrained from adding the "time dimension" to the event of returning their call.

An hour had passed by, and now Kuru was pacing up and down the hall. Suddenly he stopped as though struck by lightning. "I have lots of doctors in my family in Kolkata. Someone should be able to shed some light on this," he muttered and picked up the phone.

"Kuru, it is three in the morning in India right now. Wait for an hour at least," Ninjja said.

"My uncle wouldn't mind if I woke him in the middle of night for this," he said with a deep breath as he settled down in the sofa.

The reticent housekeeper could sense that something was amiss, and she did the best that she could do in that situation: served them piping-hot Indian ginger tea.

Kuru went in to get the prescription and started making a mental note of all the symptoms that he felt were important to describe. Their preparation was interrupted by Ninjja's sister, who sauntered in with the gait of a person who had crossed the line of sobriety. The disturbing sight underscored the need for some sort of urgent action, and without brooding any further, Kuru bolted into the next room to make his call. Ninjja had to control her urge to be an active participant in the discussion and instead decided to focus on her sister.

Her caring "Would you like to eat something?" was met with no response at all. There was no point in getting annoyed, so Ninjja made the decision herself and served some food that she believed would appeal to her sister.

To her pleasant surprise, the food was devoured in no time, and the second helping also met with a similar fate. The housekeeper tried to conceal her surprise at this newly demonstrated appetite and looked the other way.

Ninjja wanted to change the mood in the room and made a stealthy attempt by switching on the TV. She was relieved to see that her sister didn't object to the TV but was actually staring at it. In short order, the baby also joined the party, completing the "ladies' quorum."

•   •   •

Ninjja couldn't suppress her curiosity anymore. Kuru was in the process of thanking his uncle and saying good-bye when Ninjja walked in with a big question mark written all over her face. "Your guess was right. Medicines are playing havoc with her." Kuru continued cautiously, "The side effects of drowsiness, confusion, loss of balance and motor control, increased appetite, and so on are all fairly common with such a high dosage. Some people also suffer nausea, rashes, or some other extreme behaviors like delirium. The good news, though, is that the impact is temporary if one doesn't take this medication on a long-term basis."

"What should we do in this case?" Ninjja was relieved to know that they were not at the extreme end of spectrum, yet the information wasn't enough to alleviate all the anxiety.

"Gradually reducing the dosage along with resuming normal chores is the only solution. To my uncle, the dosage seemed very strong, but he was not in a position to recommend anything," Kuru responded.

Ninjja's eyes lit up. "Now we have pointed questions that we need to ask our doctor. We need to clearly describe our observations and ask if these are indeed the side effects, or if something is really wrong with the patient. And ask about the plan for reducing the dosage."

"Yes, of course. Let's hope that we get to speak to the doctor soon enough." Kuru did not sound too hopeful. "However, before we do anything else, I need to make it up to your sister for snapping at her for no fault of hers," he said remorsefully. The guilt and sorrow that Ninjja saw on his face really moved her.

· · ·

Time was running out.

Now Ninjja had less than twenty-four hours to go before her flight took off for India. She started reviewing the basic facts of the situation:

- Staying away from work for too long was not a recommended path for career progression.
- The doctor had indicated no reasons for worry during his review.

- There was a housekeeper in place to take care of basic chores, and within two weeks, her parents would be in a condition to fly down and lend a helping hand.

To sum it up, all the technical parameters supported Ninjja's return journey.

Later that evening, their attending doctor also called back and acknowledged that the steroid dosage might have to be tinkered with. He also reassured them that there was no reason to worry as long as the patient was not moving about unattended. Ninjja saw this as a sign of final approval for her return. She gathered herself with a heavy heart and initiated the process of packing up.

• • •

Ninjja's sister was slowly absorbing the events around her. Ninjja was feeling very low, but there was no better time to return home. As Ninjja was throwing the last few pieces of miscellaneous items into her suitcase, her sister sat beside Ninjja's luggage and pleaded, "Can you take the baby with you? I am scared. I don't know what will happen to her if you are gone."

Ninjja was taken aback. "What are you saying? Kuru is such a good father. Nothing will happen to your baby." Ninjja had to overcome a sinking feeling to muster these few words.

"I am good for nothing; how can Kuru possibly manage everything?" She looked up pitifully and managed to voice her thoughts after a long pause.

Ninjja couldn't muster any reaction other than silence. She was scared to look at her sister, who had tears in her eyes.

Finally, Ninjja's sister broke the ice by coming closer and giving her a tight hug. There was a heartrending silence for next few minutes. Ninjja felt that she would choke under the avalanche of emotion that was building up inside her.

None of the technical factors had any relevance for her decision making any more. In a split second, she had found her voice back and whispered, "You need to move now. I have to call the airline to postpone my ticket." The statement registered almost instantly, and the surprised bliss that she saw on her sister's face was a treasure that Ninjja would never trade for anything else in life.

. . .

Kuru, who had been trying to hide his nervousness all evening, looked much more at ease as he settled down in front of the TV. To their surprise, Ninjja's sister joined them and started chatting. She had transformed from her sedated, drunken state to her normal cheerful self. Ninjja was glad that if nothing else, her decision had acted as an antidote to the steroids, at least temporarily.

She was happy that she had actually allowed emotions to cloud her decision. If everything were just rational, perhaps we wouldn't hear of any people taking on the world for love, no stories of someone risking his or her life to save someone unknown, or of someone giving up everything for an innovation.

. . .

She was yet again amazed by the simplicity of her parents. Her sudden decision to come to the United States, their negligible conversations with her sister, and now Ninjja's decision to extend her leave by another week should have rung an alarm bell in any worldly wise person. While Ninjja was often upset at how others took advantage of her parents' naïveté, on this particular occasion, she saw this as a blessing that actually made her make-believe stories stick. Given their weak emotional disposition, the double catastrophe that the truth could have led to was enough to send a chill through her spine. The fact that her parents had led a normal life so far made her believe that even in today's complex world, goodness still prevailed.

The day had numerous ups and downs with some dramatic outcomes. Ninjja felt the need to share it with someone neutral and found herself dialing Arv's number yet again.

• • •

"Hello, stranger!" she heard the welcoming voice on the other end.

Even before she could start her dialogue, Arv stole her thunder. "Actually, I was thinking of calling you last night. I have a serious issue to discuss."

"All right, you go first, then," Ninjja replied nonchalantly. She was confident in betting with herself on what the issue might be.

"Remember the pretty Sikh girl I had mentioned to you some time back?" Arv sounded impatient for her response.

"Hmm…is this the one with long hair?" Ninjja asked, trying to jog her memory.

"Yeah…it looks like she is really interested in me. Yesterday she almost pushed me to propose. I managed to somehow deflect the issue." Arv was now speaking at a higher pitch.

"OK. I see. It doesn't feel like this is something new. You woo a girl; she gets interested; you get cold feet and then want to escape."

"Well…*no!* Things are different this time," Arv protested vehemently. He continued, "I think she is really beautiful. She is fun-loving and good to talk to. Other men are envious of me…I think…I like her."

For a change, it did seem that Arv was still interested in this woman (even after she had fallen for him). Ninjja was unable to spot the issue as yet.

Arv's monologue was still on. "After the incident yesterday, when I thought about it some more, I realized that this was also a perfect match with the kind of daughter-in-law that my parents want…she is tall, fair, and not a doctor or an engineer or an MBA; she wants to be a homemaker, loves tradition, and has one older brother. Her father is…"

"OK, OK, *stop*." Ninjja burst into uncontrollable laughter. "Are you saying that your parents have prepared a detailed specification sheet that you need to comply with?" After catching her breath and ignoring Arv's annoyed grunts, she continued with amusement, "This is hilarious. I can't believe that such a checklist could be prepared at this level of detail."

"You can laugh as much as you like after I put the phone down," Arv snapped.

"OK, OK, I am sorry." Ninjja tried to control her amusement and continued with some sensitivity, "Look, I don't see if the situation can be any better than this. You have always maintained that you would never marry someone your parents didn't approve of. How can anything be better than this? I just don't see where the problem is."

"Exactly. If I take this proposal to my parents, they are going to be ecstatic. There is no chance in hell that they would say no. So I need to be two hundred percent sure!"

"So what's stopping you from being two hundred percent sure?" Ninjja quizzed him further.

"Well…I have known her for just six months, maybe…she is nice, but there are a few things that I don't necessarily enjoy. She loves to shop…fashion, dressing up and looking good is extremely important to her…she doesn't enjoy sports, she doesn't like adventurous travel, and she expects me to be chivalrous all the time! What if I can't put up with this after I get married?" An element of concern was evident in Arv's voice now.

Ninjja was amused, but she continued to handle the sensitive topic with as much care as she could. "Arv, what you have just described sounds pretty normal to me. These are the traits of any normal girl, and you'd better learn to accept it."

Arv was in no mood to relent. He argued, "You don't have any of these characteristics, so how can you justify this as a normal girly thing?"

Ninjja had to bring out her armor. " I had limited exposure in my small town…and if you add the influence of a prudish convent and an austere mother, the word "fashion" was not even in my vocabulary. When I grew up, I studied and worked in places where there were hardly any women. Where was the opportunity to develop girly habits? Or maybe I am fundamentally abnormal—I don't know!" Unintentionally, she sounded abrupt. She regained her composure and continued, "Let me make this easier for you. Look at the other women you know—your other friends, your cousins, your mother, your aunts, past girlfriends you have had. Don't you see these features as common threads?"

There was long pause at the other end. This insight had struck Arv like a thunderbolt. He was amazed at how he had missed something so obvious. He resumed slowly, "OK. I understand...I was wrong! But...however normal this might be...I think it will still annoy me."

Now it was Ninjja's turn to get annoyed. "Get real, Arv! The world is not perfect, and no human is perfect! If you want to add all of your likes and dislikes to the specifications that your parents desire, you'll need a custom-designed human, and you'd better start looking for options in a laboratory!"

"I am sorry. I didn't mean to irritate you. But the fact is that I can't decide. I really don't know what to do."

The sincerity in Arv's tone helped Ninjja soften her approach.

"Arv, first of all, I think you should stop ticking off a checklist and listen to your heart. I have no right to claim any expertise on this topic, but I am offering my two cents, since you asked for it. Please ask yourself if this person adds new energy to your life. Would you be devastated if this person walked out of your life right now?"

Her voice seemed to come from far away—she had gone back to her old roommate Tina. Tina was continuing to tick off the checklist that society had given her. A biannual visit to an Ashram and secretly taken antidepressants were helping her to be just fine.

"Arv, are you there?" Ninjja was back from her reverie.

It seemed like Arv was also lost somewhere in parallel.

"Yes, I am here. I heard you. You have got me thinking. OK, tell me what you wanted to talk about."

"Oh, nothing major. We can talk about it some other time. I have delayed my return journey by a week—that's all." Ninjja had lost her enthusiasm to discuss the events of the day.

. . .

Ninjja settled down on the bed beside the baby's bassinet. The baby looked so peaceful that Ninjja had an impish desire to test the soundness of her sleep. She gently laid her finger on the baby's palm and waited for a reaction. The baby smiled in her sleep, and before Ninjja realized it, she had grabbed her finger. Ninjja tried to wriggle out gently, but the baby whimpered in protest.

Ninjja made one more attempt, but the sound of protest grew louder. Just the thought of having to handle the full-blown howling scared Ninjja so much that she happily pushed her finger back into baby's tiny fist and waited for things to settle down. Within a few seconds, the baby went back to the status quo of peace, except that Ninjja's finger was stuck inside the bassinet!

Mentally rebuking herself, she pulled her arm over the bassinet (with her finger still firmly in the small fist) and tried to lie down on one side. It was a difficult but not impossible posture to sleep in.

. . .

Ninjja woke up in acute pain. She tried to find her bearings and traced the source of pain to her unsupported arm that was still hanging inside the bassinet. It was three in the morning. The pain was so bad that there was no time to be afraid of the howling.

After half an hour of nursing her sore arm with an icepack, she felt a little better.

The small incident had taught Ninjja an important lesson: *Don't mess with a sleeping baby!*

On a more serious note, she understood the value of patience. *Sometimes, even a small, innocuous incident can create disturbance in the body. One needs to give it appropriate time and attention to recover.* If an unsavory sleeping posture could create so much trouble, expecting her sister to start behaving normally within a span of few weeks was indeed ludicrous. She vowed to display more patience and sensitivity as she lay down to sleep again.

Six

The Unfinished Agenda

As always, mornings reminded Ninjja of the unfinished agenda at hand. She was glad that she was able to cut through the blur that the statistics on enormous leakage had created in her mind.

She collected different pages where she had scribbled her thoughts. She went on to the next step of laying out the actions that each category of stakeholders could take independently to improve health-care delivery to the poor (details of which can be found in the pages from Ninjja's diary in Appendix 2).

Clearly the Good Samaritans like the global welfare organizations, charities, and governments were in an excellent position to promote a healthy collaboration between the private players and the donors, link funding to outcome or results metrics instead of the input parameters (as is done mostly), force transparency, prioritize prevention, push enabling regulations, and so on.

The poor themselves would need to take on responsibility for their own well-being by taking advantage of free preventive health checkups, being conscious of sanitation standards, creating a personal health-care corpus, and so on.

The employers in the informal sector can also play an important role by spreading awareness about "value of health" and supporting the poor in becoming health-care enabled.

Lack of education among the underprivileged compounded the challenge, but Ninjja was confident that a "viral method" of spreading the message could work.

She took an example of an average urban household in India. The underprivileged people in the informal sector that the household comes into contact with regularly are plenty: at least one maid, one garbage collector, the guard of the building, the lift operator, the building gardener, the building sweeper, the rickshaw puller, and so on. Clearly, the list is not short. It wouldn't be wrong to assume that the thirty-five million middle- and high-income households can potentially influence one hundred million households or more.

Fortunately, most of these poor in the urban centers still have their roots in the rural areas and are now well connected to them— thanks to mobile telephones. Adding a multiplier effect of just one for their rural counterparts, they could touch another one hundred million households! Suddenly, this shrinks the whole country without the need for an elaborate budget and bureaucracy.

At the minimum this could help address the bottleneck of awareness, which is the first step for any systemic change. The only things that are needed are social conscientiousness and will.

· · ·

"Where are you, lost?" Kuru interrupted her rigorous, brain-churning activity.

Ninjja welcomed his intervention. Like a quintessential Bengali, within five minutes, Kuru was actively engaged in her deliberations.

"There is a fundamental flaw in your logic," he opined.

"What do you mean?" Ninjja was completely rattled by this sudden rejoinder.

"You don't have to go very far. How many people do you see littering the streets from their cars? Haven't you noticed people dropping garbage on the street just a few meters away from their fancy homes? How many people use substandard vehicles or adulterated fuel, leading to air pollution? How many people eat heavy meals late at night?"

Ninjja's eyes had widened with this new perspective, but she let Kuru continue his dialogue. "The chances are that all these people are from the urban educated class. Unfortunately, they don't appreciate the link between general sanitation, our eating habits, lifestyle, and health." Kuru was now riding a train that had no brakes. "How many people do you know who have complained about doctors' consultation fees being too high? They would happily pay five hundred rupees [ten dollars] for a haircut or a beauty treatment, but when the same amount has to be paid to get health-related advice, it is considered exorbitant…this is your social conscientiousness!"

"Hmm…understood! Education does not equal health awareness!" Ninjja stopped as though defeated by the harsh reality that Kuru had just portrayed. However, she bounced back relatively quickly. "OK, we need to go back a few steps and then…the first line of attack needs to be these thirty-five million households, and the rest will follow. The good news is that these people can be accessed through multiple modes: corporate initiative, media, social forums, etcetera…" Ninjja's eyes had lit up again. "And by the way, not everybody falls in the 'blissfully unconcerned' category. While we do notice the people littering from their cars, there are plenty who don't. The 'already converted' can kick-start the process without waiting for any external aid."

Kuru had been listening intently. Now, it was his turn to have the final word: "I can see a ray of hope. The challenge is difficult but not impossible."

"I agree. Challenges are never easy. We all know that after the disastrous famines that killed millions, it took more than three decades of 'green revolution' to increase the cereal production threefold and feed the growing population in India. The health situation at hand doesn't need anything less than a revolution. If we want to reap the benefits, the magnitude and intensity of the effort has to be much higher."

"The good news is that compared to the situation in the sixties, we are now armed with three things that can accelerate the change: better literacy across strata, connectivity (mobiles and TV penetration has made everyone accessible), and confidence that individuals and private enterprise can also make a difference (and it is not only for the government to bring about change). Even if we start with a handful of people who have a strong will and conviction to pass on the determination to few others, we would have won half the battle."

Kuru was now beginning to appreciate the positive strokes in an otherwise grim situation. "I like this concept of 'viral method' and your optimism! Let me make a beginning by talking to at least three friends." Kuru's tone was definitive as he walked toward the main door to answer the doorbell.

Ninjja was feeling satisfied and was thankful to Kuru for challenging her thinking. However, the satisfaction wasn't enough to satiate her craving for breakfast. She found her feet automatically turning toward the kitchen.

•   •   •

As she turned her attention to the for-profit market participants like hospitals, pharmaceutical companies, insurance companies, medical equipment makers, and so on, it became more difficult to identify the compelling logic that would encourage them to serve the poor. Although focus on prevention made sense from the perspective of all the other stakeholders, it was questionable when it came to the for-profit players. *Why would any business enterprise take an action that cannibalizes its own business?*

Unhealthy lifestyles and growth in diseases seemed like good trends for most of the for-profit players.

Can these market participants continue to grow their profits till perpetuity by just focusing on the narrow segment (treatment for the well-to-do) that they have chosen now? Shouldn't "prevention for all" be the new mantra? Ninjja wondered.

She started reviewing some basic facts to assess the feasibility:

- The incidence of diseases and disease-related deaths was highest in poorer countries, supporting her notion that the poor and the prevention both were ignored.

- With an increase in wealth, the incidence of communicable diseases decreased dramatically (potentially due to improved living conditions, better awareness, and access to health-care); however, other lifestyle diseases, such as heart diseases, problems related to obesity, depression, sleep disorders, and complications associated with overmedication, started taking over.

Her hazy memories of the medicinal habits of several of her American friends suddenly started coming to life for her. Susan, Mary, Mike, Jack…all had one thing in common: their day started with a healthy dosage of pills, followed by several S.O.S. (medical abbreviation for 'if needed') medicines. They all had very good reasons: "This one is for general wellness," "This one is for immunity," "This one helps me sleep during flights," "Oh, this one is just 'Ty,'" "This has no side effects," "This is a wonder drug that helps me when I have long, hectic days or less time to sleep…"

No wonder the per capita expenditure on OTC drugs in the United States is almost twice as much that of Japan (despite Japan's much older population) and three times that of Germany or Denmark. Ninjja was now able to connect her observations with statistics.

Switching her attention to the well-to-do people around her in India, she realized that there were enough people who bestowed the same honor on pills as one normally would on popcorn during a movie. Furthermore, there were plenty of doctors who loved to write enough prescriptions to suck out all the ink in a pen, lest there might be an ailment that went unattended.

The patients and the health-care providers both competed on this issue. There were patients who had no tolerance or patience to cope with minimal external stimuli. Similarly, many doctors measured their success with the speed at which they could get a patient up and running.

Access to treatment combined with fast lifestyles created a mind-set of "a pill for every problem" and diverted attention from prevention or lifestyle management.

Ninjja was concerned as she extended this phenomenon into future. What would happen when these well-to-do people grew old and didn't have the ability to pay from their pocket for the OTC drugs? Would these habits lead to more serious ailments that shift the burden from the individual to the state or to the insurance company?

Clearly, the governments, insurance companies, and individuals concerned stood to lose in such a scenario.

Maybe higher-intensity medical care worsened the productive life span for even the privileged class instead of improving it, thereby reducing their wealth-creation potential. Additionally, the lesser-privileged people would get further alienated, creating a downward spiral of minor ailments that could catapult into health catastrophes. Even if a country had a strong social-security system to pay for everyone, ultimately, the inability to generate enough wealth would catch up and lead to a complete collapse of the system.

The United States was a case in point—the widening gap between health-care funding requirements and the availability of funds had already started manifesting in the form of a budget squeeze, higher copays, tighter norms for cost of treatment, and so on. The pain-sharing across different constituents would only magnify if dramatic corrective steps were not taken.

Keeping the moral and ethical principles aside, increasing the profit pool through more and more expensive procedures and treatment methods deployed on the same narrow segment (that would likely get narrower) didn't look feasible over the longer term, even on pure economic principles.

Either the health-care machinery could depend on governments to take money away from other deserving categories of expenditure (e.g., education, infrastructure, etc.), or it needed to expand its scope.

• • •

Ninjja came back to reality with a jolt that was delivered to her in the form of a smoke alarm. The housekeeper had decided to make a really potent curry that meant smoking the oil and decimating all the good ingredients that the spices may have possessed before incineration.

While this might turn out to be appealing to the taste buds, it certainly didn't go down well with the alarm system installed in the kitchen. To spice things up further, an uncontrollable coughing bout from her sister accompanied by the cranky crying of the baby took the ensuing chaos to a completely new level.

• • •

Back in her thinking chair, Ninjja was relieved to find that there was still some hope in a prima facie bleak situation.

While the temptation to focus on short-term returns at the cost of longer-term peril was not new, keeping one's eyes shut to impending doom would be foolhardy. Inventing new models to serve other segments would become necessary—if not out of benevolence and philanthropy, then at least out of self-preservation.

For-profit participants could take a proactive approach to PPP (public-private partnership) to expand the available market and bring in the much-needed efficiency in the system, focus their efforts on prevention and create new innovative products and so on. The funding agencies could provide the much-needed financial support to make the economics work. Even if only 10 percent of leakage of a total US $6.5 trillion health-care expenditure could be plugged through the involvement of the private sector, better controls, and so on, suddenly funds upward of US $650 billion would become available to support the subsidy, changes, and innovations required.

They could also attack the cost curve by focusing on "minimum sufficiency." Several industries like mobile phones, TVs, cameras, and cars had transformed themselves from "eclectic" to "mass market" by focusing on the cost curve.

She wondered why such a revolution was not visible in health-care and wrote her closing thought in her diary: "If we are not seeing such dramatic changes in health-care, it is potentially not because of design but because of choice. The good news is that necessity can force the choice to change."

• • •

Seven

The transition

It was time for Ninjja to head back. Even if one knows something is inevitable, the emotional response to a situation cannot be predicted. An otherwise composed Ninjja was feeling completely disoriented and distressed as her sister and brother-in-law drove her to the airport. Surprisingly, her sister demonstrated incredible courage and came along to the airport to see her off.

After going through the routine of the check-in process, Ninjja proceeded to the circus of the security check. The little mercy that it offered was that visitors were allowed to accompany the passenger till the entry point. The queue was long, but Ninjja was not complaining as it allowed her the opportunity to have her sister and the little baby in sight.

Ninjja took her time removing her shoes, belt, jacket, and laptop in a surreptitious attempt to steal few more extra minutes with her family. Once reunited with her belongings coming out of the X-ray machine, Ninjja turned back to get one last good look at her sister. Ninjja waved her hand with all her might, fully aware that given her sister's eyesight, she must be seeing only a hazy image of her from that distance.

Her sister continued to wave back in the same general direction (duly guided by Kuru) as Ninjja started slowly moving backward toward her boarding gate. A good twenty meters of walking backward seemed relatively easily under the circumstances.

.   .   .

Once at the boarding gate, she settled down in an empty corner chair and started waiting for the boarding announcement. Suddenly, Ninjja was feeling purposeless.

The time slowly slipped by, and once they boarded, Ninjja found herself being herded to her seat. Her expectations were so low that she considered herself extremely fortunate to get the last corner seat that had three inches of extra space on the side. The sight of a personal screen was an added plus. After the takeoff, Ninjja picked a comedy film to watch, but she couldn't get into the mood to appreciate the humor. She switched to flipping through the in-flight magazine, but nothing could fill the emptiness that she was experiencing within. Listless, she decided to close her eyes and started anchoring her thoughts on her eager parents and the work that awaited her.

.   .   .

Ninjja woke up with a jolt and panicked. She felt like she had dropped the baby from her lap. It took her couple of seconds to realize that she was on the plane, and they were passing through a high-turbulence zone.

The vigorous movement had sent her hands flying away from her lap, creating a hybrid reality-dream sequence. Ninjja noticed that people around her were also in panic, albeit for a different (and real) reason. Shaking food trays and falling cups and glasses could hardly be considered a minor, passing trouble. Ninjja was still feeling dazed and looked around with a blank expression. The general panic on the plane lasted for at least five minutes, giving Ninjja enough time and stimulus to find her bearings.

She slept for the remainder of the journey, with a bizarre backdrop of the feeling that the baby was still sleeping on her lap.

. . .

In the wee hours of the morning, when Ninjja reached home, a bout of nervousness hit her. She would no longer be able to hide the truth from her parents. The time for unfolding the whole picture was staring at her.

. . .

Over next couple of days, Ninjja was glad to find that she had underestimated her parents. They absorbed the news in a rather composed manner. Ninjja wasn't sure whether this was due to a sudden transformation in their mind-set or just the fact that Ninjja wouldn't have come back if there were still a crisis. Irrespective of the reason, she was relieved that the difficult task that she was dreading so much had passed off rather smoothly.

Except for a disoriented sleeping pattern, everything else seemed normal. Ninjja would often wake up suddenly and panic when she didn't see the baby sleeping there. Sometimes she would perfunctorily get up to make milk and then realize that she was now in a different place and time. This was a new discovery for Ninjja. Unknowingly, her brain had ingrained certain new, reflexive actions so deeply that even repeated reminders about the changed reality did not have much of an impact. *Wow, looks like the movies are not all that unreal. If without any conscious effort my brain has gotten trained for these new reflexes, then surely with focused effort, it is possible to train and condition one's brain to achieve the unthinkable!*

Amazed by the complexity and potential of the human brain, Ninjja started thinking about ways to untrain her brain as she tried to resume her sleep.

● ● ●

Ninjja was annoyed with the sound of a ringing bell in the background. She was hoping that the ringing would go away, but it refused to stop, forcing her to acknowledge it as emanating from her phone. "Hello," she responded groggily.

"Hello, darling. If you are thinking that I am disturbing you at four in the morning, you are slightly wrong," her friend Uma said on the other end.

"Oh, what time is it?"

"Ten o'clock in the morning," came the reply. That was enough to spring Ninjja out of her bed in a split second. "Gosh, I am so damn late for work. I will talk to you later…and thank you for the wake-up call." Ninjja was mad at her parents for bestowing their usual kindness yet again on her to let her oversleep.

"I tried, but you looked so tired…you were not responding…" Her mother offered a lame excuse that Ninjja summarily dismissed in the ensuing rush.

. . .

"There is some good news. I can actually see you off till Singapore for your US trip!" Ninjja exclaimed in a chirpy mood later that evening. "So stop worrying about the wheelchair and changing terminals and millions of other problems that you have been imagining."

"I don't get it. How is this possible?" asked her mother.

"I have been asked to go to Singapore for work for two days, and I have chosen the same flight as yours. Does this make sense now?"

Suddenly the ambient conditions in the room changed dramatically. It looked as though a crushing weight had been lifted off her parents' chests. Ninjja was able to appreciate the full magnitude of stress that they were experiencing only after she could see the amount of excitement that replaced it.

. . .

SEPTEMBER 2007

With the storm that had hit her family now below the danger mark, Ninjja had started resuming her regular life. She was on a task that was duller than dusting a house—a thorough review of footnotes (typically written in font size seven and probably not read by even the authors) on each slide of the one hundred page presentation sitting on her desk—when Arv called her with a strange request.

"Hey, listen…I have two free tickets to Singapore that are going to expire in three weeks. Will you come with me?" Ninjja's eyes widened with surprise, but even before she could react, Arv pushed his way through. "Kush, Veer, and Shaan are all tied up. Please, please,

please, don't say no…it's perfect timing…I know that you also have a valid visa!"

"Of course you know that…I just got back and told you that the consulate benevolently gave me a five-year multiple-entry visa this time. That doesn't mean I should start holidaying with you. What happened to your several million girlfriends? I am sure someone is going to love this trip. How about the pretty girl with long hair?" Ninjja blurted out the last sentence without thinking and then bit her lip, wondering if she had accidentally touched the wrong chord.

Arv was unperturbed. "You don't understand. It is complicated. Everyone does not have the independence of making their own decisions, "especially girls"! That's really hard."

"And who do you think I am? By the way, I don't think independence is given by someone…you need to take it," Ninjja snapped.

"Yeah, whatever…what matters is that we are going to have loads of fun!"

"Oh, hello! Don't start putting words in my mouth. I never said yes. I have truckloads of work piled up for me. Besides, it would be silly to go back to the same place within a few weeks. My colleagues are going to think I am out of my mind." Ninjja tried to take control of the discussion but failed miserably.

"OK…tell me, what have you seen besides your hotel or the offices that you have visited for meetings? And the airport, of course," he added sarcastically.

"Why does it matter? The city is a business center! Give me a break, for God's sake," Ninjja responded peevishly, for lack of a better answer.

"OK, let's see. From the little that I know, this place is a shopper's paradise, it has a vibrant nightlife, the riverside restaurants are…"

Ninjja interrupted loudly, "Can we drop this, please? I have work to do."

Arv took notice and moved over to another topic. Finally, when they were about to hang up, Arv dropped a subtle hint: "We can discuss this again later."

After dinner, when Ninjja settled back in her bed with her laptop, she felt a shooting pain in her wrist. She had been experiencing a subtle pain for several months now, but the one today was interfering with her comfort.

With every keystroke, the pain seemed to increase, and every click of the mouse felt like a mild electric shock. The physical constraints curtailed her enthusiasm to continue with work for next few hours.

Overnight rest helped. Ninjja chose the easier path of considering the issue as a passing ignorable phenomenon, with the naïveté of a child who believes that he is invisible to the whole world if he closes his eyes.

• • •

Finally, the weekend shopping trip she'd planned with Uma was happening. In passing, Ninjja mentioned the offer of a free Singapore ticket to Uma, and she got all excited. "I think you should go," Uma started off in a sermonizing tone that Ninjja often dreaded.

"Are you out of your mind? How on earth can you even think that this is possible?"

"Arv is right; it will be worth visiting Singapore once as a tourist. Wouldn't you have come with me if I had asked you to come?"

"That's different. Also, it would depend on the timing."

"Why is it different? Isn't Arv a really good friend who stands by you in your hour of need? Don't you trust him?"

She paused for a second and then, as though struck by a flash of insight, she pounced on Ninjja with a mischievous glint in her eyes: "Wait a minute..."

Irritated, Ninjja cut her off. "I simply don't have the time. It would be stupid to ask for leave when I have just gotten back from a long, personal emergency...let's go to another shop." Uma sensed that the temperature was raging high and embraced silence as her best friend at that moment.

Later that evening, Arv had a new value proposition for her: "Here is a plan. A three-day weekend is coming up in two weeks. You won't have to take any leave. Also, there are some good hotel deals, if one books two rooms at one shot. You can just join me for meals if your work can't wait. What say you?"

Given the difficulty in getting one's preferred dates on free tickets and at short notice, Ninjja considered the chances of success as next to nil. This was her opportunity to get Arv off her back without having to actually go with him.

"Fine. Let me think about this." Ninjja left the conversation open-ended.

"That's great; let me check on the booking dates…you will not be able to escape if the booking gets confirmed."

"I would die if I were to plan so much," Ninjja muttered to herself as she disconnected the call.

• • •

Ninjja was in a meeting with one of her senior colleagues when he suddenly changed the topic of discussion. "What's wrong with your hand?" Ninjja looked around to see if he was referring to someone else in the room, but she didn't spot any other recipient of his attention.

He noticed the confused look on Ninjja's face and continued, "You have been constantly squeezing your hand. Looks like there is some severe pain. Don't ignore it. It might be due to the computer. I know of people who had to quit their jobs because the problem became very acute."

"Oh, no, there is nothing serious. I am sure it will be fine tomorrow. It has its own cycle of cropping up and going away…I will keep it under watch. Thanks." Ninjja tried to divert the attention from her back to the topic that they were discussing.

Ninjja was indeed alarmed with the severity of the consequences that he'd just described, but she rationalized to herself that her senior colleague had a well-deserved reputation of being an exaggerator.

. . .

A text message from Arv distracted her: "Tickets confirmed."

"Oh, no! I can't believe this is really happening!" Ninjja mumbled as she headed out from the meeting room.

The next week flew by very quickly with the pressure to ensure there was no spillover of work to the weekend. Ninjja wasn't entirely sure of her feelings for the trip. As she was packing her bag, she was oscillating between excitement and some unknown apprehension.

To save herself, she chose to ignore the occasional guilt pang for pushing some of the "nice to-do" work to an undefined timeframe.

. . .

As always, she pushed her luck to the limits to reach the airport at the last minute. While collecting her boarding pass, she was nervous about Arv's ridicule that was awaiting her. Arv, the superplanner, had been waiting there for two hours and was just waiting to attack her.

Once inside the plane, Ninjja got her opportunity for revenge. The excitement of getting the emergency row evaporated rather quickly with the discovery that the seats were nonreclining and did not have the extra leg space that often goes with the emergency row.

"I never knew that they could have nonreclining seats on international flights! No wonder you got the preferred dates at such short notice on a free ticket! This is unbelievable." Ninjja started her teasing spree. "Why on earth did you travel so much on this airline to earn a free ticket? Beats me completely."

The airhostess, who looked as dilapidated and tired as the plane, came by to provide the standard discourse on actions needed during an emergency landing. After the ritual was over, Arv tried to hide his embarrassment. "Look, the good part is that we have an empty seat on this row…learn to value the horizontal space also."

"Yeah, little mercies. I am glad that the person in the middle seat managed to find another spot. Good for him, and good for us!" Ninjja retorted.

Carrying her laptop bag and the luggage had aggravated the pain in her wrist. She was inadvertently pressing some painful spots while trying to sleep.

Fortunately, the hectic activity of the day combined with the insipid food had the much-needed numbing effect to put her to sleep.

· · ·

The flight was about to land. Ninjja had totally forgotten about her wrist, as the neck pain due to her bad sleeping posture became the focus of her attention. To Ninjja's surprise, Arv appeared (or pretended) to be totally fresh and full of energy. He did not want to lose the opportunity of making fun of Ninjja's recent health hiccups, so he resumed his banter: "Will squeezing your neck help in relieving the pain? I will happily oblige."

. . .

This time around, the city looked very different to Ninjja. A drab business city seemed colorful and vibrant. *Can our mind-set make so much of a difference in how we perceive the same thing?* Ninjja asked herself, but she restrained herself from expressing these thoughts to Arv, for obvious reasons.

Arv went out of his way to find a good vegetarian restaurant for Ninjja, despite a clear signal from her that she would be happy to survive on potatoes and salad. Ninjja hadn't noticed this part of Arv's personality before. He had a caring side to him behind all his tough-ness and sarcasm.

Once they settled down, Arv posed a difficult question: "Why do you always have some body part troubling you? Stomach issues, gid-diness, knee pain, back pain, wrist pain...this is where my knowledge of biology ends...but all I can say is that the list is fairly long."

"It is probably due to the long hours at work and little time to rest. Nothing used to happen during my school and college days. Despite gobbling pastries and puffs every day, my stomach was fine, and I never put on weight. Do you know that my mother's side of family is full of healthy nonagenarians? I used to think that my strong genes would always carry me through...Guess their impact is waning now," Ninjja responded casually.

Arv remained unimpressed. "I also work long hours and several of my friends in investment banking have an even tougher life. We don't have such an assortment of health issues." He continued to push for the root cause. "By the way, whenever I have heard you talk about your childhood, I have heard of pastries, samosas, puffs, and the like. Did you ever eat normal food?" he added sarcastically. As the discussion progressed, Ninjja found a deep contrast in their growing-up years. She had hated fruits, vegetables, and milk, thereby ignoring vital nutrients. Sports and outdoor activities had been a big no-no. To top it all, her overanxious parents found even the slightest health hiccup a reason enough to get medical attention for her.

While Arv agreed that it was impossible to pinpoint an exact root cause, the differences were enough to make Ninjja sit up and take notice.

"I suspect that you would have been in worse shape if it hadn't been for your strong genes," Arv said in his final caustic remark.

She was intrigued by this discovery. Once back in the comfort zone of her room, she settled down to do her own research to find out if some of these differences in the formative years made such a big impact all through her life.

What she discovered was a big eye-opener. The impact of early life diet and lifestyle on future health seemed to be a hot topic among researchers. Given the difficulty in isolating all the other conditions and following up with the same sample over a lifespan, it was hard to create a statistical correlation. However, there seemed to be no dispute about the fact that early stage lifestyle (active versus inactive), environment, and intake of nutrients played a critical role in future health. Though it was not impossible to make up for some of the shortfall, recovering fully from lost development in the early stage was nearly unfeasible.

She stared wide-eyed at some of the findings of the researchers:

"Genes and experiences interact to determine an individual's vulnerability to early adversity and, for children experiencing severe adversity, environmental influences appear to be at least if not more powerful than genetic predispositions in their impact on the odds of having chronic health problems later in life.

When these systems are being constructed early in life, a child's experiences and environments have powerful influences on both their immediate development and subsequent functioning. These effects may appear early and be magnified later as children grow into adolescence and adulthood. **Some have compared a child's evolving health status in the early years to the launching of a rocket, as small disruptions that occur shortly after takeoff can have very large effects on its ultimate trajectory.** Thus, "getting things right" and establishing strong biological systems in early childhood can help to avoid costly and less effective attempts to "fix" problems as they emerge later in life." (Center on the Developing Child at Harvard University, "The Foundations of Lifelong Health Are Built in Early Childhood" [working paper, 2010], http://developingchild.harvard.edu/resources/reports_and_working_papers/foundations-of-lifelong-health.)

There was no way for her to go back to her early childhood and correct for some of the glaring mistakes in eating habits and lifestyle that had occurred due to her parents' pampering and her own brattish behavior.

Shockingly, the mistakes in her upbringing were driven by lack of awareness rather than actual scarcity or affordability of a balanced diet and lifestyle. *There must be so many other children who might be ending up undernourished and will suffer health issues through adulthood in spite of having the means. How can we have people end up with poor health due to bad choices for lack of awareness?*

Ninjja was baffled to realize that it wasn't only economic status that drove the issue of malnourishment—lack of awareness and the luxury to exercise choices could be equally dangerous!

She rushed to get her yellow diary to jot down her learning. She wished she could communicate her own experience to every child and parent that she could find! She wondered if all the preschools and schools could have a mandatory class for parents on the do's and don'ts for a balanced lifestyle for their child and the severity of consequences that might unfold as she picked up the pen.

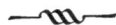

My Survival Mantra

1. Don't assume that your regular physician will always know what is right for you
2. When in doubt, seek a second opinion.
3. Always have health insurance and carefully select the plan.
4. Don't rush to a specialist based on your perceived issue.
5. A balanced lifestyle holds the secret of many a cure.
6. In situations of emergency (e.g., an accident), don't run to the closest hospital.
7. If someone dear to you is admitted to the hospital, don't assume that the nurses and attendants are always right

8. Several diseases may have stress as the underlying cause.

9. Watch out for medicine addiction!

10. Emotional support is a substitute for some medicines.

11. Don't take medicines in blind faith.

12. There is no utopian health-care system.

13. **Childhood nutrition and lifestyle define a large portion of adult health**: If one has the means to spend adequately on food, there is no excuse for not creating a balanced diet and lifestyle for one's child in the formative years. As is the case with values that are mostly acquired in childhood, the foundation of good health is laid in the early years of life. Ask yourself if you really understand the meaning of a balanced diet for your child and how much physical activity is needed. A focus on child nutrition should also form the most critical part of the public-private initiatives discussed earlier for the economically backward sections. If we believe that better health of a nation's people drives the health of the nation, this aspect should deserve attention at least equal to, if not more than, that needed for creating the health-care infrastructure.

—m—

It was high time she caught some sleep, as there was a hectic schedule with the details of every fifteen minutes worked out for the next day. As per Arv's plan, they were supposed to be out and on the streets by 8:00 a.m. sharp. "He should have been in the army. Any woman who decides to marry him will need a lot of best wishes to survive!" Ninjja grumbled as she switched off the lights.

•   •   •

Ninjja's luggage had multiplied itself just to the limit that would not require any extra charge from the airlines. The deep-discount season had unshackled any restraints that Ninjja might have trained herself to follow while shopping.

"You came here with an almost empty bag, and now you have two bulging ones…I never knew you were capable of this," Arv commented jokingly.

"I can't be blamed for hoarding for the next two years, if I can get better quality, a lot more choice…and at half the price that I normally pay!" Ninjja smiled back. "However, I don't think my wrist and shoulder have taken this extra weight kindly," she continued as the shooting pain from her wrist had now reached the elbow and also the shoulder and the neck.

•   •   •

Back at work with renewed energy, Ninjja and her senior team were testing their meeting-management skills to drive a client discussion toward a decision. Unfortunately, success remained elusive. When the meeting ended, out of exhaustion rather than conclusion, Ninjja couldn't stop wondering if time had become an infinitely available resource that was being abused so callously. Last she checked, the day still had twenty-four hours. Considering seven to eight hours of sleep for a normal human and two to three hours for commuting in a big city, less than 60 percent of the day was available to split between work, self, and family. Clearly, something needed to take a backseat.

The obvious choice for most would be to deprioritize personal time and family time, as most people recognized their performance targets at work, while responsibilities toward self and family remained free of any targets and measures. The innumerable stories that she had heard from top executives about not being able to find time for their hobbies, not being able to be with their wives when they were delivering their first child, not being able to be with ailing parents, and so on corroborated her theory.

She wondered if anyone had studied the second-order effect of such a constant tension on an individual's health. Cutting the meeting time by half through focus and discipline had the potential to release at least two hours per day on average. Ninjja had no statistical data to prove this, but based on the combined experience of her coworkers, she felt comfortable with her conclusion. For an economy that was couple of trillion dollars, this would be no less than billions of dollars!

The intangible value of reduced stress and increased personal time for family, self, or attention to health could exceed the monetary value manifold. Was she getting obsessed with the issue of well-being?

She was reassured as she remembered a Sanskrit saying that she had heard in her childhood: "आयुष: क्षण एकोपि सर्वरत्नैर्न लभ्यते |नायते तद् वृथा येन प्रामाद: सुमहान्नहो (Even if you surrender all the wealth that you possess, you will not get back a single second of the time that has passed away in your life)." Yet she could not contain her bewilderment with corporate India's lack of respect for the wisdom of their own forefathers, while there was a dogged focus to learn the best practices of management from the West!

She hoped that as a nation, they would start treating time as a scarce resource, along with the long list of natural resources like oil, water, trees, and pure air. Only then could the country move to the right orbit of well-being.

● ● ●

One week later, Ninjja was struggling to do even her daily chores with her right hand. The simple tasks of holding a pen or turning a doorknob had turned painful. At this point, Ninjja had to stop and take notice. The ostrich formula wasn't working anymore.

To her surprise, the doctor told her that, unlike most of the pain she had experienced earlier, this one was not muscular but related to the nerves. Due to the long hours (and possibly incorrect posture) on the laptop, one of the nerves had gotten stressed. Pinching of the nerve at various points was causing the pain. The doctor assured her that ten physiotherapy sessions were all that she would need to get back to normal.

● ● ●

Two months later, Ninjja was religiously following the exercise routine and still going for her physiotherapy sessions, but there was no improvement whatsoever. Her right hand was now incapable of holding anything or even writing. On the positive side, Ninjja did not need to write any notes during the meetings. Delegation had become her favorite tool.

Till this happened, Ninjja hadn't realized that one needs to think even more clearly when one is dictating to someone rather than writing oneself. As with every negative event comes something positive, so it did with this disability. Ninjja learned the art of delegation and clarity of thought, and, on the physical side, she had become relatively ambidextrous.

Despite all these positives, operating without her right hand occasionally sent some chills down her spine. After following her doctor's advice for what seemed like long enough, she decided to go for a second opinion. The diagnosis remained the same, but the solution suggested was indeed dramatic.

After patiently hearing her case history and doing his own examination, the doctor professed, "You have pushed your problem too far. There is nothing beyond this that can be done with physiotherapy. Given that now the pain has reached points near the spine, we will need to look at surgical options."

Ninjja was taking everything in very calmly and was about to ask about the time for recovery when the doctor decided to go to the next step of explaining the procedure: "To release the pinching, we will need to open up the spinal area and then fix the nerve that is creating the trouble."

This was enough to send Ninjja into a full-blown panic. Just the mention of opening up something as critical as the spinal cord sent many scary thoughts racing. *What if they touch the wrong nerve? What if something else goes wrong? I might get crippled for life!* She tried to keep her outside appearance look calm and thanked the doctor for the valuable information that he had shared with her. She rushed out, gasping for breath and completely crestfallen. She dialed Uma's number, but nobody answered the call. "Madam must have gone to her meditation camp," Ninjja muttered, and she went on to call Arv. For once, she didn't give him any chance to speak until her side of the story was finished.

"Calm down! No one is opening up your spine tomorrow. You have time. Go for a third opinion…fourth, if need be…before doing something so drastic," Arv responded, helping her regain some of her lost composure.

Ninjja started her search for finding the right doctors for a third and fourth opinion. The only way to get names was by talking to people and hearing stories that established the credibility of these doctors.

During one such conversation, one of her colleagues mentioned to her that a man who was not a medical doctor had cured him of his chronic back pain. "What are you saying? How did you take such a risk?" Ninjja remarked in disbelief. "We are not even talking about an institution that practices alternate medicine…this is a one-man show who doesn't even have a clinic space and does home visits to treat patients." Ninjja's surprise grew as she learned more about this man.

Given the other drastic option that was staring at her, she decided to meet this person at least once before writing him off.

The next day, a short, stocky man with a dark complexion and a heavy regional accent showed up right at the agreed time. He had a clerical job at a government organization, which partly explained the luxury of spare time that he had.

He mentioned that he had learned his healing technique from a Chinese doctor who was practicing in India several years ago.

As Ninjja started describing her symptoms and the pain points on her arm, he patiently listened with an occasional nod and mumble. A few minutes later, he surprised Ninjja by asking if the pain had already reached certain specific points on the back and shoulder as well as on the collarbone. Ninjja had assumed that the pain on the collarbone that had come up recently was an unrelated event with no connection to her arm whatsoever. This new discovery caused as much alarm as it gave comfort that at least he understood her problem.

The prognosis of this unofficial healer was the same as that of the medical doctors: there was some sort of pressure on the nerves. Fortunately, the solution he suggested didn't involve any physical cuts.

Considering that there wasn't a plethora of happy options for her treatment and that the downside risks appeared to be much less in comparison to the potential upside, Ninjja decided to give this modified version of acupressure a shot.

Her purported healer got to work immediately. A combination of knuckles, fingertips, and a pointed, penlike device attacked Ninjja's aching right arm with full gusto and left her completely breathless.

After regaining her balance, Ninjja felt a throbbing pain that was absolutely incompatible with the beaming smile that her healer bore. He sensed her confusion and tried comforting her. "Today, it will hurt more, but tomorrow you should feel better."

Ninjja was mortified at the thought of facing the wrath of the regular physicians and desperately hoped that his words were true.

After twenty-four hours, the pain was still there, but it was at a level that was low enough to give Ninjja the courage to go for the second session.

Four weeks slipped by. The original estimate of the healer on the number of sessions needed was far exceeded. However, the trend was encouraging enough for Ninjja to continue her treatment.

Three months later, Ninjja had regained the strength in her right hand, and the pain had retreated, only to resurface when abused with long hours on the laptop. Ninjja knew that she had to manage the situation carefully and started following the discipline of right ergonomics, usage of an external mouse, and strict adherence to exercise interspersed with work.

Needless to say, her problem was not 100 percent cured (or curable), but it was at a healthy balance that would allow her to continue her work without much discomfort.

This was a living proof of the experience that she had heard from a fellow passenger during a flight. Alternative therapies existed, yet knowledge and credibility of them remained suspect. There was no easy answer on this topic, yet there was a meaningful lesson that Ninjja didn't want to lose after the trials and tribulations of the past year.

— ᴍ —

My Survival Mantra

1. Don't assume that your regular physician will always know what is right for you.
2. When in doubt, seek a second opinion.

3. Always have health insurance, and carefully select the plan.

4. Don't rush to a specialist based on your perceived issue.

5. A balanced lifestyle holds the secret of many a cure.

6. In emergency situations (e.g., an accident), don't run to the closest hospital.

7. If someone dear to you is admitted to the hospital, don't assume that the nurses and attendants are always right.

8. Several diseases may have stress as the underlying cause.

9. Watch out for medicine addiction!

10. Emotional support is a substitute to some medicines.

11. Don't take medicines in blind faith.

12. There is no utopian health-care system.

13. Childhood diet and lifestyle define a large portion of adult health.

14. **Explore alternative therapies before going under the knife if you are not in a time-critical situation.** At times, traditional medicine has its limitations, and invasive procedures and surgery become the only options available. It is important to understand whether one has the time to explore alternative options; and if the answer is yes, an earnest attempt to identify the alternatives should be made. Though the paucity of information makes finding alternative therapies difficult, it should not be considered any harder than finding the right path in the mainstream approach, where the

abundance of information (quantity rather than quality) becomes a stumbling block. In alternative therapies, testing the credibility through word of mouth and meeting actual patients as well as assessing the risks of a certain treatment should help in making the right trade-offs. When choosing the alternative route, watching out for quacks should become an integral part of the due-diligence process, as accreditation mechanisms are weak compared to the mainstream approach. Once the decision to pursue an alternate treatment is made after appropriate due diligence, the progress and signals of any risks need to be watched out for carefully. Interestingly, some of the alternative therapies could be continued in parallel to traditional medicine, and there are examples of success through a combined model.

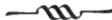

Eight

The Unthinkable

11:00 P.M., AUGUST 2009

Ninjja was startled by the loud ringing of her phone. Her heart skipped a beat, as the number on the caller ID was that of her parents' neighbor. *Oh God! Why are they calling? At this hour? Hope all is well at home.* Millions of scary thoughts crossed her mind in a split second as she reached for the phone.

Ten minutes later, Ninjja was sitting frozen in her chair. She was trying to replay the conversation in her head...but it still seemed surreal. Probably, the mind has its own cycle time of recovering from shock and numbness. Half an hour later, she realized that doing nothing was not the right answer. Something didn't seem right. It was pretty late at night, but fortunately it was midday in the other part of world. Ninjja called up her sister in the United States, who was surprised to get her call at an odd hour. She heard the story in disbelief and went through similar emotions.

Perhaps the secondhand narration subdued some of the intensity. "There must be some misunderstanding," her sister finally said. "I guess we will need to wait till tomorrow to resolve this."

Ninjja was not happy with this answer. There was something amiss, and the discussion with her sister was not helping her find it. "Why do you think they didn't call at an earlier time?" Ninjja tried to put forward one of the pieces that didn't seem to fit. But the discussion kept getting more entangled, potentially because both the parties were more emotional than rational at this stage. Finally, they decided to speak again in the morning and hung up.

Ninjja was still disturbed. Her brain, which was trained to come up with hypotheses for solving every problem, seemed to draw a blank. In desperation, she dialed Arv.

"Arv, I am really sorry to bother you so late...but I need to talk." Ninjja's voice had a mix of apology and a plea that immediately caught Arv's attention.

"You don't need to be sorry. I have a critical deliverable due tomorrow, so I was up in any case. Tell me what's bothering you."

"It is odd...I don't know how I should say this..." Ninjja paused for several seconds and then continued, "I can't believe any of this... this is so bizarre..."

"Ninjja, these riddles are not going to help. I have absolutely no idea what you are talking about. Can you please get to the meat straight away?" Arv said in a commanding tone.

"Um...I received a call from my parents' neighbors late, around eleven o'clock. They want me to come down to resolve a situation. This concerns my father." Ninjja had to pause again. She was trying to muster the courage to say the unthinkable.

"They are claiming that he has been misbehaving...they are talking of improper behavior with children!"

Now it was Arv's turn to be shocked. "What!" He couldn't find another word after this.

Ninjja had gathered her strength again to continue. "Is it possible? Can a perfectly honorable septuagenarian suddenly lose his mind and start indulging in such activities? Believe me, he is actually so simple that some folks call him saintly!" Ninjja continued on for the fear of hearing silence on the other end. "He is a man of extremely high integrity!" Ninjja kept speaking as though trying to seek justification in her own mind. "He is a dedicated husband and a perfect dad, and he's probably the most gentle person that I have ever seen...this cannot be true..."

Now, Ninjja seemed to be talking to herself, and Arv was in no position to utter a word. The monologue continued: "I haven't heard anything odd from my mother, nor did I notice anything strange when I met him three weeks ago...can only one part of wiring in the brain suddenly go wrong? To be honest, I didn't know how to react to this kind of conversation. I tried to probe a little despite my shock and dismay." Ninjja paused for breath and went on: "When I asked about how and when they got to know about this, they claimed that it has been going on for three years. Isn't this odd? Why did they wait for three years?"

There was a brief pause, and then Arv found his speech back: "Hold on! Just tell me everything from the beginning. Who are these people? How exactly did they start the conversation? What is their relationship with your parents? How well do you know them? Keep your emotions aside, and please tell me all the facts."

It was hard for Ninjja to disengage herself from the devastating allegations, yet Arv's authoritative tone helped her gather herself. She started rattling out the facts in random order: "The call came from two of the neighbors...the two men claimed that they were waiting for rest of their family members to retire for the day before calling me. They said that, given the supersensitive nature of the dialogue, they couldn't speak when others were around.

"They mentioned that they had not confronted my parents out of concern for my father's health. When questioned further, they had added that they refrained from reaching out to my mother for the fear of hassling her.

"My parents have known these neighbors for the past four years (since the time they moved into this new area). I used to end up meeting them (not necessarily by choice) every time I visited my parents. They seemed very friendly and helpful to my parents..."

Ninjja paused briefly as though trying to remember if she was omitting anything important. Arv didn't want to interrupt her flow and maintained the utmost discretion. Soon enough, Ninjja resumed: "When I first saw these three little girls, they were between two and five years of age. They used to pop in any time they felt like and used to love playing with my parents..." As though feeling a need to put some context behind these events, she added, "Just so you know, my mother is a retired schoolteacher! She genuinely does enjoy educating the little ones! The drive for meaningful occupation and the feeling that she was contributing to the formative years of these little children was so strong that she never cared about any remuneration...and she taught them for free.

"Also, my father is a great storyteller. I have often seen him regale these children with his fantastic tales. Overall, this seemed to be a happy arrangement for all concerned."

Ninjja put forward her main conclusion. She was about to stop, when couple more things struck her. "Ah, and a few other things," she continued. "Since the past year, two other kids from the neighborhood have started taking lessons from my mother, and they are showing great progress! I don't know these other kids well, but I think these two men mentioned the name of one of these new kids also as a victim...strange, isn't it?

"During this call they kept pushing me to come over there to discuss and settle the matter with them. Does this give you enough of a background?" Ninjja paused finally for Arv's reaction.

Arv, who had been taking in all this information with rapt attention, was itching to ask some more questions and jumped in immediately: "You didn't tell me anything about the occupation of these two friendly neighbors."

"I think the next-door neighbor works at a government department as a clerk, and the one who lives opposite our house is a small-time dealer of a consumer goods company," Ninjja answered, straining her memory.

"Do they know that your dad needs psychiatric treatment to manage his cycles of depression?" Arv quizzed her again.

"Umm…I am sure they know it. My parents' life is an open book. But why does this matter?" Ninjja was perplexed.

"For now, just keep answering my questions. I will explain later." Arv was in no mood to waste time in consensus building and fired another question at her: "Did these neighbors ever ask for any financial help?"

"No," Ninjja replied immediately, and then she stopped as though struck by lightning. "Well, now that I am thinking…I can say that there weren't direct requests, but certainly there were some insinuations! Surely, some convoluted ideas were presented to my parents that would have entailed financial gains for the neighbors." She stopped, trying to remember the details.

Now Arv's voice bore curiosity: "Tell me more…what was the nature of this discussion? How did it end up?"

"About a year ago, the neighbor offered to construct a floor in his house where my parents could move in instead of living in the current rented house. For some reason, my parents seemed to like the idea. I think the cost estimate that the neighbor gave was about ten lakhs. I vetoed it, as the land rights looked fuzzy, and I didn't want to wrack my head over it." Ninjja took a deep breath and continued, "My dad was telling me a few weeks ago that the neighbor was asking him to invest in a farm, but my dad had no interest…" Ninjja thought a little more and then slowly recollected another incident: "I can think of another discussion about six months ago. This is the time when the neighbor was trying to buy a car. He had called me to seek my advice regarding a loan. He mentioned that he was facing some issues regarding the loan approval. I could think of a technical solution and had suggested it to him. Do you think he was expecting some financial help?"

Now, Ninjja could sense where Arv was going with his line of questioning. The process of exploration was throwing in new insights, yet Ninjja was not ready to believe this direction.

"Can't you see what is going on? There is nothing wrong with your dad. Here is a doting daughter who will do anything to protect her father. The father is vulnerable, as he suffers from depression. That makes the situation even more perfect for a conspiracy to extract ransom. It is so easy…no need to go through the trouble of kidnapping…just create stress and get a handsome payoff."

Arv didn't get any reaction from Ninjja, prompting him to continue proving his case: "Why didn't they go to the cops instead of calling you? They know that you wouldn't want them to harass your father, as it is unlikely that he will be able to handle it. Ninjja, think a little harder about your conversation with them. Can you find any other supporting arguments for this theory? Are there any holes in the story they told you? The allegation that they have come up with is extremely serious. We need to have a game plan in place before tomorrow morning."

Ninjja's earlier shock was now replaced by a new jolt of betrayal. Was it possible that someone who was trusted like a family member could hatch such a plan?

Ninjja was even more concerned about her father's safety and well-being than she had been during that ominous call. She tried to take control of her emotions and started testing the hypotheses that Arv had just floated. "Arv, your theory is worth testing. Now that I think about this, I can see that there are several things about this call that look odd in hindsight. Let me start off with some top of the mind things.

"The reason to call me so late at night is not convincing enough. Were they trying to scare me? Isn't it odd that two men decided to call me regarding such a sensitive topic rather than the mothers of these children? If indeed there was an issue, it would be fitting for women to have a chat with a woman, given our societal construct."

Ninjja was feeling baffled and enlightened at the same time. She continued to rattle out odd facts: "Probably they were not prepared for my question on 'When did you get to know?' and blurted 'Three years' to show the severity of the situation. They'd need to be totally out of their minds to let their children spend four to eight hours at a neighbor's house when they had doubts. How atrocious can this be!

"When I told them that I would discuss this with my mother and ask her to speak to them, they were not too happy. They kept pushing me to come down to have a discussion with them and to not bother my mother…the word 'settle' was used way too often. It could have been a euphemism of 'financial settlement.'"

As Ninjja kept talking, she was struck by another discovery. She couldn't believe that she had completely missed the subtle threat during the call.

"They had mentioned that the parents of the new student were so upset that they wanted to thrash my father…and that these two gentlemen had done us a great favor by managing the situation and were now giving me the opportunity to settle the matter."

Now it was Arv's turn to give a cry of surprise. "What! How could you skip something so vital in your story? Can't you see the subtle threat? Don't you think this squarely supports our theory of a conspiracy? The reason they called you late was to catch you unawares and ensure that you didn't have any time to discuss this with anyone. They wanted to scare you enough so that you took the first flight next morning.

"The allegation that they have chosen is so serious that just an innuendo from the children would be enough to initiate criminal proceedings. Your neighbors know that the consequences on your father's physical and mental health would be devastating. They probably presumed that you would get so anxious that you would concede to any financial demands that were within your limits." Arv was now speaking in an agitated tone. He was excited that he was getting closer to a conspiracy theory that seemed to be watertight, yet nervous that there was no easy solution on the horizon.

Ninjja still couldn't believe what she was hearing. She looked for reasons to poke holes in this theory and started challenging Arv: "They were always so friendly and caring...just few months back, they bought gifts for my mother as a token of their gratitude after the school results."

"With this backdrop, doesn't the call now look even more fishy?" Arv stopped her counterargument midway and continued, "If these children were being troubled for the past three years, then one can't be any less than a god to forgive and shower gifts on the perpetrator of such an evil. Clearly this scheme was concocted after the school results."

Relentless as she was, Ninjja did not want to leave any angle unexplored. She continued, "Why now? Why did they wait all these years? "

It was already past one o'clock, yet Arv was displaying remarkable sharpness and aplomb. He continued, "Ninjja, a devious plan is neither instantaneous nor planned for eternity. There has to be a compelling reason, and the timing needs to fit in. From what you described earlier, it seems their income is just sufficient for normal sustenance...given the ever-expanding expectations of today's world, a financial need is not too farfetched to imagine. Didn't you mention the difficulty that the neighbor was facing in getting a car loan? Isn't it clear to you that he was spending beyond his means? Your gullible parents were possibly sitting ducks to target."

Ninjja listened intently to this compelling story that Arv was weaving with the facts that she had rattled in random order.

"Clearly, finding a motive is not that difficult. Now, let's come to the issue of timing. Haven't you bought an apartment recently in a posh building?" Arv's unrelated comment caught her unawares.

She remembered how excited she was four weeks earlier after getting the loan approval for her dream apartment. "What does it have to do with this situation?" Ninjja asked him.

"I am sure that you shared this happiness with your parents," Arv replied. "Considering their open-book policy, I am sure that the neighbors knew about it." He stopped to see if there was any reaction from Ninjja.

Now, it was Ninjja's turn to jump in and complete the missing part of the story: "Are you saying that this piece of information convinced them that this was the perfect time to squeeze some cash out?"

"Exactly! Now you are thinking like a criminal!" Arv finally gave a sigh of relief.

Ninjja found his logic convincing enough to at least accept it as their working theory and think ahead.

Arv went on, "How deep is this conspiracy? Are some other people also involved? Were they just making up the story about the new kid, or are his parents also part of the conspiracy? Do they have some support outside in the legal system to execute their plan?"

Arv's trail of questions seemed never-ending. It was evident that prudence was his number-one priority, and Ninjja was glad that he was able to think about the worst-case scenario.

Ninjja had recovered her poise now and made an attempt to support Arv's thinking process to her best abilities. "This is a good question. I don't know. The parents of all these kids seem to be good friends...and I really can't say how deep the conspiracy is. If we were to assume that this is a game plan of just these two neighbors, with no friendly support from someone within the law-enforcement agencies, then things should be manageable. In this scenario, one could take them head-on (with help from the statements of the new students). Hopefully, the fear of public shame would force these neighbors to recoil. However, in the worst-case scenario, things could turn out to be really ugly and potentially endanger my father's life." Ninjja found it difficult to control her emotions again and broke down. "What if all of them are involved, and they barge into my parents' house with cops? My father will be definitely taken in for questioning…he may get a severe attack of depression. Just the humiliation will kill him…by the time the truth is discovered, it will be too late! Arv, there is no option! I will need to shut them up!"

Fortunately, Arv's thinking was not clouded with emotion. "What if your parents are evacuated from there before these schemers get a chance to act? The only thing you need to do is to buy some time!"

This new approach completely surprised Ninjja. This was the first time that she had experienced the meaning of "out-of-the-box" thinking in real life. By two thirty, they had a solid defense plan in place.

• • •

Ninjja managed to send off her parents to her sister's place in the United States within forty-eight hours of receiving the threatening call. She kept the neighbors engaged in the meanwhile with excuses like, "Couldn't get the flight ticket…I am trying my best to come over…give me another day."

Her aunt and uncle, who lived in the same vicinity, played an important role in helping her parents get out of harm's reach. She was glad that her whole extended family stood by her father, without an iota of doubt.

Once the conspirators realized that their target had disappeared, their true selves bared their ugly teeth. They started calling Ninjja incessantly, and when she didn't pick up, they walked across to her aunt's house and abused her profusely. This was followed by a series of nasty e-mails that provided additional proof of the conspiracy. The inconsistencies across various statements and the desperation in their tone became more obvious.

As days turned to weeks, the calls tapered away.

Arv had helped Ninjja to be mentally prepared to deal with the situation, just in case the conspirators decided to turn up at her doorstep. Fortunately, the occasion to exercise her well-rehearsed response did not arise.

. . .

Ninjja was glad that the episode was finally over, and the conspirators had to accept defeat. Success in such a situation required presence of mind, meticulous planning, execution, and strong willpower from everyone involved.

While the extreme-scenario thinking did save her parents from direct harm, the trauma that they had experienced was no less. Her sister had to constantly counsel them to help them forget the deceit and move on. For simple, trusting individuals, it was not easy. Even the antics of her cute little niece (who was now two years old) could not divert their attention fully. The sting of betrayal is worse than the one given by a deathstalker, a dangerous species of scorpion whose sting is extraordinarily painful.

. . .

With time, the wounds were gradually healing.

It was a relaxed, late evening, and Ninjja was engaged in a friendly banter with her sister, who suggested, "I think you should write a thriller based on this experience. There are many ways this episode could have unfolded, and it is our good fortune that we managed to survive without many skeletons on the way. Every senior citizen could learn something from this."

Ninjja parked the idea of writing a crime thriller for later, but she couldn't help thinking about the social challenges and exploitation that one can get exposed to due to health-related issues. There was something worth penning down in her yellow diary after this grueling experience.

Her root-cause analysis pointed to one thing: "A philosophy of full transparency with all works either in the ideal world or, for the audacious, in the real world."

She had a strong belief that if the conspirators had known about the financials but not about her father's psychiatric treatment and vulnerability, this devious master plan could not have taken shape.

She was not unaware of how people with certain diseases were ostracized, but a criminal conspiracy where a person's health was used as a primary weapon was new to her. Out of curiosity, she started reading about this topic and found many intriguing and scary stories.

She was compelled to turn to a new page in her diary.

My Survival Mantra

1. Don't assume that your regular physician will always know what is right for you.
2. When in doubt, seek a second opinion.
3. Always have health insurance, and carefully select the plan.
4. Don't rush to a specialist based on your perceived issue.
5. Overseas insurance is not a blank check.
6. A balanced lifestyle holds the secret of many a cure.
7. In emergency situations (e.g., an accident), don't run to the closest hospital.
8. If someone dear to you is admitted to the hospital, don't assume that the nurses and attendants are always right.
9. Several diseases may have stress as the underlying cause.
10. Watch out for medicine addiction!
11. Emotional support is a substitute for some medicines.
12. Don't take medicines in blind faith.
13. There is no utopian health-care system.
14. Childhood diet and lifestyle define a large portion of adult health.
15. Explore alternative therapies before going under the knife if you are not in a time-critical situation.
16. **Think before you start making all your health issues public:** Talking about health problems to get sympathy and support from people

around you is a common human behavior. However, be aware that some unscrupulous people may try to take advantage of your weakness. The range of such deceit could vary from simple things, like taking undue favors, to finding an innocuous way into your will, to loathsome methods of extortion, kidnapping, blackmailing, and so on at the extreme end. This danger of manipulation may multiply if you are a senior citizen who is perceived to be financially sound. Some discretion to differentiate between what should be public information versus private is necessary for self-preservation. Follow some simple rules of thumb to protect against any probability of falling prey to such a scheme. Rule 1: there is no need to broadcast physical or mental disabilities (especially if they are not visible to the naked eye). Rule 2: keep the doctor-patient discussions confidential; only your inner circle of people needs to stay informed. Rule 3: it is important to demonstrate that you are not dependent on anyone around you.

Nine

X-Rayed

MARCH 2010

Ninjja's parents were now living with her after facing the hurtful treachery of their neighbors.

She had changed her job and was all excited about the career jump that came along with it. She was thoroughly enjoying the new responsibility and challenges, but as an inadvertent downside, she could spare even less time for her family.

Single-day business trips that offered her the luxury of sleeping in her own bed turned out to be far more energy-sapping than she had imagined. She had totally underestimated the unwelcome adventures due to increases in airport security, perennial renovation at the airports, and lack of infrastructure and skills to manage even a slight sneeze of the weather gods. The only positive flicker in this madness on the social dimension was that being on the road from five in the morning till about midnight created plenty of chance meetings with her long-lost friends.

However, by the time she got back home, her father would be in a deep sleep. It was ironic that being under the same roof did not translate into even meeting every day. Ninjja was trying hard to convince herself that this was fait accompli, and there was no need to feel guilty.

How do women with children manage this lifestyle? Hats off to supermoms! Ninjja thought with awe and disbelief as she dropped onto her bed with a thud.

Why am I just thinking about women? Don't children need their father as well? She chided herself for thinking of the stereotypes. *Are all of these successful professionals indeed superhumans, or have they learned to take this trade-off as a fait accompli as well? The chances of these superhumans being able to control timeliness of flights or to control the road traffic seems next to nil. My earlier thinking of managing meetings efficiently is going to help only in finding personal time but is not going to solve the problem of failing to see one's family when the job demands crazy travel.*

This dialogue with herself helped her get over her guilt temporarily; she found solace in the fact that she did get ample opportunity to chat with her parents during her long hours in traffic jams. "Thank God for mobile telephones!" Ninjja muttered as she fell asleep.

JUNE 2010

Time was slipping by, and neither Ninjja nor her parents were getting any younger. On one of the weekends, Ninjja noticed that her father's breathlessness had increased dramatically. Ninjja was aware that asthma patients were more sensitive to weather conditions, but she had no experience to judge the severity of the problem. She went by her mother's experience that such ups and downs were normal.

. . .

A few days later, her father's breathlessness had started affecting even minor chores like walking to answer the door. This was when alarm bells started ringing.

Ninjja had to travel again, but, sensing the urgency to consult a doctor, she pleaded with her parents to go to the hospital with the driver instead.

The visit to Ninjja's general physician did not result in any conclusion. The doctor wanted to see the latest X-ray report, which meant a delay of another day.

. . .

The next day, Ninjja diligently took her father for an X-ray. She was worried to see that he was unable to walk even a few feet due to breathlessness. She persuaded him to try harder, but she had to give up very soon. A wheelchair had to be called in.

Ninjja's concern had multiplied by now. However, relief would have to wait till the scheduled time of the report delivery, another twenty-four hours away.

Ninjja's anxiousness to collect the report pushed her to reach the clinic before the scheduled time. The person at the report counter asked her to wait for a few minutes while he busied himself with his regular chores.

A few minutes turned into half an hour.

Ninjja's patience was running out. At the risk of being rebuked, she went to the counter again. This time, she got an answer: "The doctor who is supposed to review the X-ray and write his report has still not come in. You will need to wait for another fifteen minutes." However, the next fifteen minutes turned into another half hour, and the X-ray report was nowhere in sight. Eventually her frustration overpowered her desire to maintain the sanctity of the clinic and manifested itself in a loud dressing down.

The report dispenser recoiled and realized that her patience had been pushed beyond its limits. He tried to communicate apologetically: "I am sorry; it seems the doctor will not be able to make it to the clinic today. You should collect the report at the same time tomorrow."

Ninjja could not believe what she had just heard. "How can you talk so casually about an additional twenty-four-hour delay in giving a diagnostic report for a potentially serious case?" she confronted him, her frustration giving way to anger. "Why don't you just give me the X-ray film without the doctor's review?"

The person at the counter was indeed trained well to be a pachyderm. After banging her head against a brick wall for few more minutes, Ninjja decided to call it a day. She was shocked at the state of affairs in one of the most reputed chains of clinics in the country. She shuddered to imagine how the government hospitals were running.

She had read about the horror stories of people dying in public hospitals due to lack of medicines, but adding a lack of timely diagnostic reports to the list of killers would not be too farfetched.

· · ·

Ninjja's parents were waiting for her for dinner and were secretly hoping that she would bring some good news from the clinic. With a heavy heart, she told them to be patient. She had to pretend that a forty-eight-hour delay (considering the doctor's visiting hours) in meeting the doctor would not have any adverse impact.

"Maybe that's why they have coined the term 'patient' for the patients...we have no other option but to be patient," Ninjja's mother lamented. Ninjja was feeling very sorry for her father, who was suffering silently.

Ninjja could not control her schedule for the next few days and had to leave her parents at the mercy of her driver for the doctor's consultation. Fortunately, the car driver she used to engage for such one-off requests was unlike the bulk of his clan in northern India—he was a well-mannered, respectful young man who followed a normal clock (and not Indian Standard Time). His availability helped Ninjja get over her guilt.

However, the news that she received after the consultation was not something that she had expected. The doctor saw some sort of a lump in the X-ray and wanted to double-check with a CT scan.

Ninjja was relieved to see that her father was taking this new development in his stride. He seemed unperturbed.

• • •

Ninjja was in an important meeting when her phone rang. She was anxiously awaiting this call. She excused herself for few minutes and eagerly awaited some good news.

"The CT scan is also showing something like a lump…so we will need to do a test to make sure it is not malignant." Ninjja's general physician was on the other end.

"Are you saying this could be cancer?" Ninjja blurted out anxiously, hoping that she was totally wrong.

"We can't rule out the possibility till we are able to take a sample. There is a procedure called a bronchoscopy, where we will put a small probe through his windpipe to view the lump and take out some tissue. It is a very simple, harmless test, and your dad will be released in a few hours," the doctor replied.

"How long can this wait?" was all that Ninjja could muster under the circumstances.
The thought of something getting shoved inside a delicate part of the body scared her.

The doctor sensed her discomfort and tried to give her the needed reassurance. "Look, just to be sure, I have also consulted the respiratory specialist. This is a completely harmless procedure and a necessary one for taking out the sample. The specialist is also here with me, and you can talk to him if you like." With no other option in sight, Ninjja took the opportunity and tried to understand the pros and cons of the proposed procedure. During the discussion, the doctors convinced her that the procedure was a must and that there was no risk. They also convinced her that delaying the test was not a good idea. Since the test had to done on an empty stomach (no food or water), the appointment was set up for the next morning.

Once Ninjja had some time to reflect that evening, she thought about the sequence of events some more. Two tests (X-ray and CT scan) and review by two doctors (one GP and one specialist) were pointing toward a "lump" in the respiratory system. Given that her father's suffering had been increasing with every passing day, something had to be done soon. Even common sense suggested that some intrusion into the body would be needed to collect a tissue from the lump for further testing.

The only question pending was the risk of the procedure. Ninjja went through the sources on Internet and found that the risks were minimal. Patients were able to leave three to four hours after the test, and only in extremely rare situations where they required to be hospitalized. To overcome her fears, she also spoke to a doctor through the referral of her friends. While the doctor added the caveat that it was difficult to comment without seeing the X-ray or CT scan, he confirmed that the procedure was generally risk-free.

Ninjja's mother was already in a panic, and Ninjja didn't think that a suggestion to delay the procedure by couple of days would go down well. Given the limitations of time, information, and mental strength, Ninjja felt comfortable with the decision that had been made a few hours earlier.

• • •

Ninjja was feeling very anxious. She kept checking on her father, despite her back-to-back meetings.

It was already noon, and the specialist had still not turned up to conduct the test. "Is it fair to keep a breathless, hungry senior citizen waiting for three hours to conduct a supposedly simple test?" Ninjja's mother vented her frustration. "None of the nurses has a clue of what is happening here."

"Maybe there are other, more serious patients who need his attention…so just relax. Dad will be fine." Ninjja tried to comfort her, knowing fully well that she wasn't a bit convinced herself about what she had just said. "Adapting rather than getting agitated would be wiser, as you don't have a choice," Ninjja added.

• • •

Two hours later her phone rang again.

Ninjja sprinted out of the meeting room to take the call. It was the specialist at the other end. He sounded full of energy and was anxious to give her some good news. What she heard next was music to Ninjja's ears: "Your dad doesn't have cancer. There is no lump. What we saw in X-ray were air pockets."

"Thank God! This is great news! Thank you, Doctor," Ninjja exclaimed. She continued, "But what is wrong? Why is he suffering so much?"

The doctor was happy to oblige and continued, "This is an advanced stage of COPD (chronic obstructive pulmonary disease)…this disease needs to be managed properly. The air pockets collapse, and then…" The long explanation vaguely reminded Ninjja of the painful, jargon-filled biology classes in school. At the earliest opportunity, Ninjja jumped in with the question that had been bothering her since the doctor had started speaking: "Can this disease be cured? How long will it take for him to feel better?"

"Well, there is nothing like a cure for this disease. As I mentioned, this disease needs to be managed well with medicines, lifestyle, and so on. Also, there is no immediate danger to his life. People with this disease can have a long life. We can discuss more when we meet. For now, you should feel happy that there is no lump. A cancer along with this kind of advanced COPD condition would have been extremely dangerous. Stop worrying. Your father is resting now. You should be able to speak to him in a couple of hours."

Ninjja concluded that the situation was serious but still redeemable. When one fears the worst, anything less than that offers relief. Ninjja was no different. She got back to her remaining meetings feeling much lighter and energetic. Ninjja hoped to see the smile back on her father's face over the weekend.

At 5:15 p.m., Ninjja was concluding her second-to-last meeting for the day when, unexpectedly, her phone rang again. Her mother was in a panic. "Your dad has to be admitted to the ICU...the hospital is asking me to deposit fifty thousand rupees [approximately one thousand dollars]. I have only five thousand with me...I just can't think...what should I do?"

Ninjja was thirteen hundred kilometers away, and even if she could take the first flight that was feasible, given the horrendous city traffic during peak hours, it would be six hours before she could get there.

Ninjja hid her turmoil and focused on the immediate task of calming her mother down. "Just stay calm. He will be fine. I will be there as soon as I can. In the meanwhile, just tell the billing desk that your daughter will settle the deposit in a few hours. If they don't believe you, just ask them to call me. I will give them my credit-card number. Is the driver there with you?" Ninjja tried to sound as calm as possible under the circumstances. She just hoped that her father was not going to add to the statistics of rare cases of complications after a bronchoscopy.

Ninjja hopped into her taxi immediately to start the treacherous journey toward the airport, while her secretary sprang into action to book the flight ticket and take care of her luggage in the hotel, along with other checkout formalities.

Fortunately, the flight was not hampered by the never-ending runway-maintenance jobs this time, and Ninjja was at the hospital entrance by eleven at night. The sight of her mother sitting forlorn in the waiting area outside the ICU was very disturbing.

Ninjja learned that her mother had not seen her dad since he was brought to the ICU. No one was prepared to give her any information.

A female guard with a strong build and attitude best suited for fierce arm-to-arm combat with an enemy met them at the main door of the ICU. Needless to say, "hospitality" was not a term that she was familiar with. Her first reaction was to drive them away. Ninjja's mother tried pleading with her and used the angle of "concerned daughter from far away desperate to see her father," with no effect.. This new character "Guardazonian" –The amazonian guard with no mercy, left her frustrated and speechless.

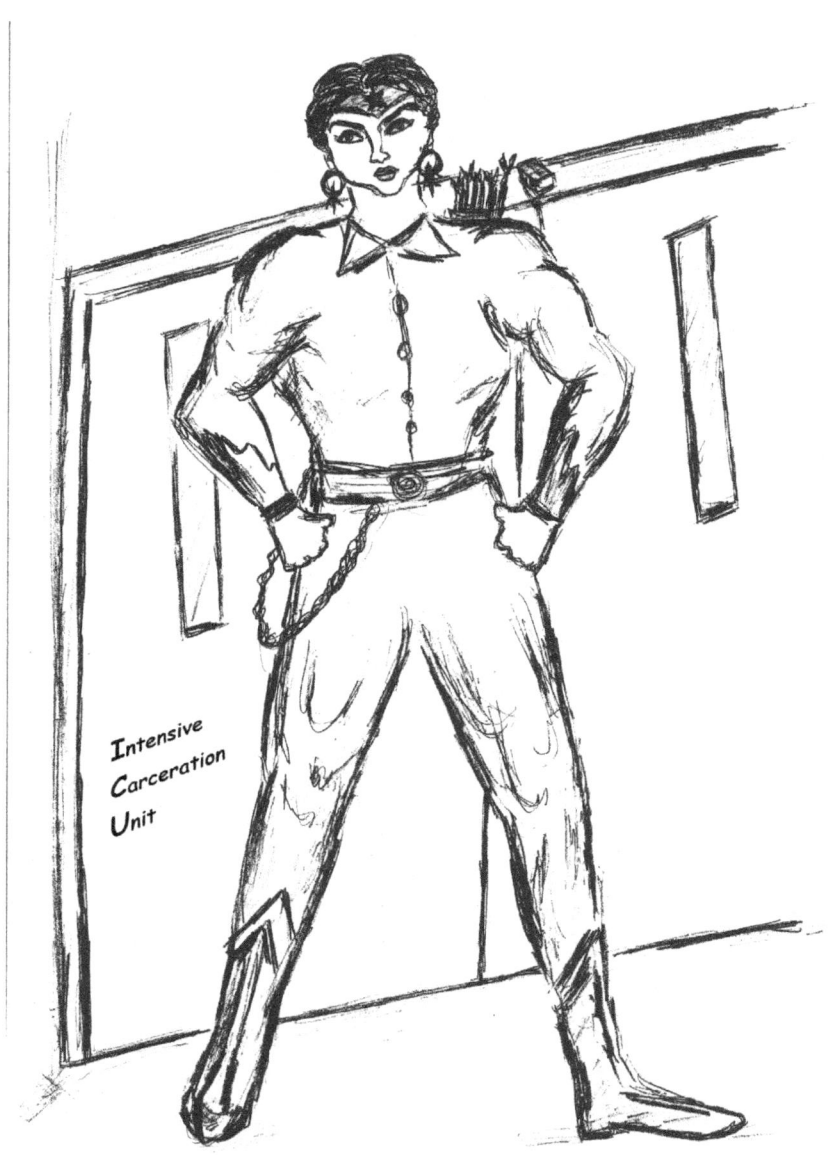

Intensive Carceration Unit

Guardazonian: Amazonian Guard who protects entry to ICU with her whole might and renders it "Intensive Carceration Unit".

Fortunately, the driver noticed a nurse walking out of the ICU who seemed familiar. He took the initiative of stopping her and realized that she lived in the same building as he did. After some small talk, he managed to convince her to allow Ninjja and her mother a five-minute visit with her father. The nurse convinced the iron lady at the gate and escorted them in.

The humming sound of various devices and machines was depressing and added to the gloomy atmosphere. Ninjja's father was sleeping with various devices attached to his body. The oxygen mask on his face scared Ninjja the most. She quickly scanned through the log lying beside his bed and was relieved to see that most of the vital indicators were fine. The nurse could not give any information regarding his status or potential release time and suggested that it would be best to wait till the doctor came for his rounds in the morning.

· · ·

The ICU had only two one-hour slots in twenty-four hours for the visitors; and for the other twenty-two hours, one was doomed to be in oblivion. And even within that one-hour slot, the complicated algorithm to control the crowd in the ICU (which was known only to the guard) ensured that one did not get more than fifteen to twenty minutes with one's loved ones. The other aspect that surprised Ninjja was the precautions that were being taken to keep the environment safe. All the visitors happily walked in with their shoes on. Even when Ninjja asked them if there were plastic shoe covers that had to be worn before entering the ICU, she was given a nod that meant no.

In the earlier era of desktop computers, a lot more precautions were taken to protect the computer room against the dust than what she saw in the modern-day ICU. In today's world, the premium real-estate model homes, which had no danger of putting anyone's life at risk, forced their visitors to wear disposable shoe covers lest there be a drop in value of the property due to lack of décor or cleanliness! It was unfortunate that it did not figure in the list of to-dos for a premium hospital.

Fortunately, the hospital had spent a small portion of per-patient income on buying comfortable chairs in the waiting area. The mother-daughter duo profusely thanked the driver before sending him off and curling up on the chairs. Sleep was nowhere in sight, but they maintained silence to preserve the slim chances of the other person getting some restful moments.

The next morning, they had a surprise visitor. One of their neighbors showed up with a flask of hot tea. It certainly did help in bringing a smile to their faces, at least temporarily.

The doctor's visiting time was still three hours away, and Ninjja was getting restless. She tried her luck again with the nurse on night duty and was ecstatic to see her dad sitting on his bed. His face brightened up with a fresh breath of life the moment his eyes caught sight of Ninjja. The joy that she saw on his face made her day.

While his physical indicators were doing better, emotionally he was feeling very lonely. "Every time I woke up at night, I looked around but didn't see you and your mother." He finally spoke after mustering all his energy. Ninjja was moved. She tried to console him by explaining the ICU protocols, but his reply stumped her: "How does that matter? I would have felt much better if both of you were by my side."

Clearly, the need for emotional support was not one of the criteria that the hospital had on its list for treating patients.

"Have you had anything to eat?" Ninjja tried to divert his attention.

"Yes, they did bring a food tray…I am not sure what it was, though." Ninjja understood the point and promised him that next time she was allowed inside, she would try to smuggle in some biscuits.

The nurse was now giving her unwelcoming looks for exceeding her time. Ninjja bid a short-term good-bye and stepped out, feeling somewhat relieved. She was unable to see any compelling logic in incarcerating her dad in the ICU. *While processes and rules are needed to run any large organization, if they alone were sufficient, companies could potentially run without any people!*

In today's world, when every company worth mentioning was talking about "EQ" (emotional quotient) as a key parameter for driving an organization's performance, shouldn't a patient's EQ figure somewhere while designing the treatment protocols in the hospitals? Ninjja wondered, as she delivered the news of her father's well-being to her mother.

A few hours later, Ninjja and her mother were called into the ICU to meet the doctor. Ninjja's dad was still sitting on his bed, looking completely exasperated. The doctor offered her the comfort that he was doing fine, but Ninjja was eager to get some answers.

"What went wrong in the first place? I thought the procedure was really simple…why did he have to land up in the ICU?" she fired off.

"These things can happen. There is nothing serious. Your dad is very weak. He couldn't handle the procedure as easily as we had imagined. Let him rest in the ICU for another day, and then take him home," one of the doctors replied casually.

Ninjja was taken aback. One did not have to be a doctor to figure out that her dad was very weak. It was obvious to the naked eye. Even a younger man would have been in poor health if he'd had to struggle for breath for the past two months. If the procedure required a certain threshold energy level, then why didn't the doctors wait for a few days to get him over the hump with medicines, at least temporarily? Why did they have to put his life at risk?

Ninjja did not want to anger the doctors, so she continued a more benign line of questioning. "Being in the ICU separates him from the family, which hurts his chances of recovery. Why can't he move to a regular private room?" Ninjja asked. She added another line as an afterthought: "Also, he has no insurance coverage, and the ICU rates are almost twice the normal rates."

The last, unplanned statement (Ninjja's experience during her mother's accident was probably helping at the subconscious level!) had the desired impact, and the doctor conceded. Ninjja continued the conversation about the future precautions, things to watch out for, and so on. The doctors happily obliged. She was told that her dad would need supplemental oxygen on an ongoing basis, and he would need to take steroids.

During the course of the conversation, Ninjja made a chance discovery. It appeared that her dad was put in the ICU not because he needed intensive care but because the normal rooms were not available. It was a shocker. The decision clearly meant a major revenue upgrade for the hospital with only emotional distress for the patient!

This was not the time to get into any arguments, so Ninjja decided to let it pass.

Once back in the waiting area, Ninjja was glad to finally see some signs of relaxation on her mother's haggard face. Ninjja left her alone and stepped aside to call Arv. She was keen to share the latest ordeal with him. She had barely started when Arv cut her off.

"What? In the ICU? It is a dangerous place. Get him out of there quickly." Ninjja dismissed his highly energized remarks as the typical Arvish reaction to anything and everything.

"You have a strong point of view on everything under the sun. Can you just relax? It cannot be all that bad to be put under higher-order care than needed…if one were to ignore the financial loss and emotional trauma for the time being."

However, Arv was unstoppable. He seemed to have stronger feelings on this topic than any others that Ninjja had discussed with him. "Trust me; I have rarely seen any old person come out of ICU in my whole extended family. It is not just the ailment that one is getting treated for that kills you…there are several other infections that one can catch. The ICU environment is not infection-proof."

Ninjja could believe this point based on her own recent observation. "Arv, please don't scare me, for heaven's sake," Ninjja pleaded.

"A large chunk of pneumonia cases occur after admission to the hospital and especially when one is in ICU...don't get me wrong. It is the most common cause of death among hospital-acquired infections and is the primary cause of death in intensive-care units. Don't rest till you are able to get him out safe and sound from the hospital. That's all." Arv stopped for breath, leaving Ninjja totally breathless.

With the silence on the other end, Arv soon realized that he had gone a bit overboard with his words of caution. He tried to mitigate some of the damage by softening his tone: "Hey, Ninjja, I didn't mean to scare you; everything seems to be on the right path. The doctors are comfortable moving him to a private room—that is the first good sign! Your dad is eating and talking—that is the second good sign! So, cheer up. Give me a call once you are in the private room. I will try to visit the hospital tomorrow."

However, Ninjja's mind was already racing ahead. Despite the exaggeration, there was some sense in what Arv had said earlier. *Doing more when less is needed can also hurt.* Ninjja could think of innumerable examples in everyday life that supported this thinking. In the health-care context, the consequences seemed even more dramatic. Overdose of antibiotics could upset the stability of the stomach and hurt immunity; an extra prick could potentially expose one to infections; a surgical procedure when not needed could leave someone scarred for life...the list was never-ending. The concept of "optimum" was not meant for just the economists or business professionals after all. She just hoped that this uncalled-for intensive care did not result in any harm in the future.

Two hours had gone by, and the promised move to the regular ward was nowhere in sight. The moratorium on meeting ICU patients was in full force, prohibiting any chances of moral support for her father. Arv's words were ringing in Ninjja's ears, and every passing minute was pushing up her anxiety index.

Ninjja had been pushed to the edge now and was compelled to raise her voice.

The guard was well trained to not understand any logic for letting the patient's family in. Ninjja kept persisting, forcing the administration in charge to pay attention. She was told to respect the hospital procedures and bear with them. However, the time for patience was long gone.

"Look, I don't know what is taking so long. Is it the paperwork, or is the room not ready? Or you don't have the staff...I don't know! At least allow me to be with my father. He wants to be with his family, and this is the least you can do. Is he being treated to get better, or is he supposed to serve a sentence for some unknown crime that he committed? I think the ICU should be renamed as the 'Isolated Confinement Unit' or the 'Intensive Carceration Unit'!"

This did move the needle a little, and Ninjja was reluctantly allowed to come in for fifteen minutes while her mother continued to wait outside.

The tug-of-war continued for another three hours before the stretcher arrived to carry her father to the private room. Ninjja offered to carry her dad's regular medicines that he had brought from home before getting admitted. The nurse curtly told her to stay away from touching any of the belongings. "As per the procedure, we will sort through everything and shift all the personal belongings to the private room. You are not allowed to carry anything from here. We will take care of everything." The nurse sounded very confident.

Ninjja had already had enough battles to fight in the last seventeen hours, so she gave in.

Finally, after a few additional hiccups (like the faulty bed in the room), the family was relieved to be together at last. The long wait combined with the rough handling during transfer had taken its toll on her father, and he was looking completely exhausted.

The promise of a small, harmless procedure had catapulted into a nightmare. To keep her spirits intact, Ninjja turned to finding nuggets of goodness in the whole episode. However, she couldn't shield herself from the bitterness that had engulfed her. "Is it a planned strategy to keep the patient's family preoccupied with procedural hurdles and delays? All the energy is easily directed toward fighting with the hospital staff, which keeps the mind away from concern for your loved one. I wonder if I should thank the hospital staff for their consideration or charge them with cruelty..." Ninjja inadvertently spoke aloud, inviting a curious glance from her mother.

Now that she had her mother's attention, she continued to regale her with more sarcasm: "The other good news is that now, you will have an opportunity to buy a new pair of shoes for Dad, as the hospital staff has misplaced his during the transfer. There is no sign that you will ever get them back. I wonder if they can have a small outlet outside the ICU that says 'We also sell shoes.'"

Ninjja's mother joined the bashing party. "And what is your rationale to justify the lost medicines? Your dad had just bought his regular lot of medicines for two thousand rupees."

Ninjja remembered the overconfident nurse who had assured her of the safe transfer of everything and reached a new level of causticity: "They are so concerned about you that they don't want you carry any extra weight when you go from here. Imagine how tiring the load of one hundred grams would have been! And in this case, they don't even need to open a new outlet. They already have one."

Their jibes were interrupted by heavy, uneven breathing sounds. Ninjja immediately leaped to her father's side. He was clutching at the BIPAP machine (equipment that adds extra pressure during inhalation and similarly supports exhalation) as if wanting to get rid of it. In a reflex action, Ninjja detached the contraption in an instant before she ran out to call the nurse. By the time she came back, her dad seemed more relaxed and was breathing evenly. The nurse dutifully went about her job of readjusting the BIPAP machine.

Ninjja's inquisitiveness did not allow her to be a silent receiver. After few evasive answers, the nurse finally indicated that the initial settings were probably too high. *Wow, another example of doing more when less is required. Why do they believe that more is better? Does it make their job easier instead of putting their experience to use?* Ninjja wondered in frustration. She had to shrug off the negativity to look after her father with a positive frame of mind.

The following day, Ninjja was hoping to secure her father's release, but the doctor remained noncommittal. Ninjja learned that he was not sure if her father would be able to breathe properly without the aid of machines. "But we haven't even tried to test his ability to breathe on his own," Ninjja argued feebly. Fortunately, the doctor paid attention and instructed the staff accordingly.

• • •

Arv kept his promise and showed up in the evening. He managed to lighten up the mood of her parents with his innumerable, nonsensical jokes. Ninjja was happy to see that her father was able to breathe with the aid of the simple oxygen cylinder and was no longer dependent on the external stimulus of BIPAP.

However, there was something that kept bothering her. When she had a chance to step out with Arv, she couldn't hold back: "There is one thing that I can't comprehend. I agree that my dad was feeling very weak when he came to the hospital for his test, but the fact is that he was walking and breathing on his own. Now, with this simple test (which should ideally maintain status quo), he has had to spend a night in the ICU and another twenty-four hours in a normal room, and he is still bedridden and dependent on external oxygen. How does one explain this? Shouldn't one get better after coming to the hospital? What am I missing here?"

Arv nodded in agreement. He paused for a moment and then replied, "I am not a doctor, nor do I have any interest in biology. However, there is one principle of science that I firmly believe in: *equilibrium*. I think, even though your dad was not well, his body was in a state of equilibrium, enabling him to function. Now that it has been tampered with, you will need to give his body some time to find the new stable state. I am sure he will get better soon. Now stop worrying about something that has already happened."

After seeing Arv off, Ninjja was still pondering over the statement that he had made. His untested theory seemed to appeal to her scientifically inclined brain as well. She prayed and hoped for the new equilibrium to establish itself at a healthier level.

Later that evening, the same mashed, dull food was served again for dinner. Hospital rules prohibited any external food to the private wards, unless it was from the hospital's own food court. The logic of "patient's health" that was offered to justify the rule seemed completely asynchronous with the quality of food that was available. Given this backdrop, Ninjja felt no qualms about smuggling in some home-cooked food for her father.

After the dinner service was over, and the nurse had retired to her cozy corner in the corridor, Ninjja pulled out the healthy and identifiable food items from the secret compartments in her bag. Dad's eyes lit up, and he proactively resumed his sitting position to devour the food quickly. As she watched him with affection, she couldn't help wondering if this was indeed a hospital that was supposed to cure people. To her, it seemed more like a prison with some latitude. The redeeming fact was that the patients were made to toil and suffer on their beds instead of laboring in the sun.

The next morning, Uma's presence gave her the much-needed confidence and optimism to hold on. The doctor indicated that supplemental oxygen was still required, hence he was ambivalent in letting him go. Ninjja recollected an earlier conversation and questioned further, "Isn't my dad supposed to use the supplemental oxygen now for life? Obviously, he can't be in the hospital all the time. Isn't it possible to make these arrangements at home? I could get a full-time nurse, if that helps! I need your help to get him comfortably settled in the home environment." Ninjja paused after her emotional plea.

The doctor nodded. "OK, if you can make the necessary arrangements at home, we can try," he responded thoughtfully.

Ninjja asked him for information on reliable agencies that could supply oxygen cylinders at home. The doctor obliged. Ninjja also learned that an alternative of electricity-based, portable air concentrators existed. This option was equally effective and more economical in the longer term. Ninjja thanked the doctor for his help and set about the task of calling different vendors.

Why wasn't this information volunteered? Was the doctor acting under some guidelines of keeping information as a trade secret and maximizing the patient's stay at the hospital? she wondered.

However, she was glad that the doctor had followed his professional ethics and given her the much-needed guidance when asked.

• • •

Within three hours, Ninjja was all set at home with the right equipment; but there was a new challenge awaiting her at the hospital.

The doctor had given the green light, and they were ready to go home. However, the ordeal of the past few days had taken a toll on her dad's confidence level. He had started displaying the same symptoms of panic that she had noticed during her sister's illness. Ninjja and her mother had their jobs cut out for the next half hour. Fortunately, the nurse on duty was very kind and went out of her way to help Ninjja's father.

It may seem straightforward, but the journey is not over till one has reached the final destination...

Soon after, a junior nurse hurriedly came in to detach various devices, remove the hospital gown, and get her dad dressed in his own clothes. She pulled out the contraption for the IV fluid (the cannula) with such force that it brutally peeled off the skin. The sight of a sizeable quantity of blood oozing out was enough to send Ninjja's dad into a tailspin. All the positive impact of past half hour of confidence building had disappeared in a split second. The only saving grace was that the nurse was petrified at her mistake and scurried to do damage control.

Twenty minutes later, things were under control again.

. . .

"Looks like finally we will be heading out," Ninjja muttered to her mother, but possibly she spoke too soon.

Ninjja had underestimated the power of the wheelchair guy. Apparently there was a shortage. Whether the shortage was of the wheelchair or of the wheelchair pusher was not exactly clear, but the net impact of the inordinate delays was becoming clearer with every passing minute. Ninjja knew that this would be enough to get her father even more tired and frustrated.

It took a good three hours after the doctor's green light for Ninjja to get back home, which was just a ten-minute drive away. Needless to say, only the hospital's discharge procedures could account for the balance time. The small test that was supposed to cost Rs.10,000 (US $200) had multiplied sevenfold.

Ninjja couldn't keep her sarcasm at bay. "Look, they knew that Dad would need to leave in a wheelchair…that's why they misplaced his shoes!"

. . .

The next morning, Ninjja's father was feeling much better. He had already accepted the new lifestyle that he was supposed to live with.

Despite his weakness and the ordeal that he had been through over the past four days, he was in reasonably good spirits. Ninjja was touched to see how comfortably he started calling the oxygen cylinder his new friend. She carefully hid her tears and went on to encourage his high spirits.

. . .

Five days later, Ninjja's dad was feeling great and had really put the painful episode behind him. He was on a high dosage of steroids that needed to be reduced gradually. At the hospital, Ninjja had checked if the follow-up consultations would have to be done with the specialist or with the regular physician (the GP), and the suggestion was to continue with either of them—it was immaterial. Given the ease of access, they chose to continue with the GP.

. . .

After ten days of gradual reduction of the dosage, Ninjja's dad did not seem to be in good shape anymore. The weather was also getting colder, and he did not feel like going out to meet with the doctor again. The phone conversation with the GP did not indicate any alarming signs. He mentioned that since the weather was getting colder, there might be some discomfort. Ninjja did not want to appear to be overreacting, so she chose not bother him again.

Shortly, the count of worried people on the ground increased by one, after the arrival of Ninjja's sister. They had a feeling that the steroid-reduction pattern had not factored in the full scope of changing weather conditions and decided to pay a visit to the respiratory specialist for his advice.

•   •   •

The reaction of the specialist was in sharp contrast to the emotions that Ninjja and her sister were feeling. He was rather cool about the situation and suggested increasing the steroid dosage. He said that this was very normal for COPD patients, especially for patients who were in the fourth stage of COPD.

Ninjja wondered if such patients were expected to suffer so badly and deteriorate so fast. "But he was not in such bad shape before he came to the hospital," she managed to meekly voice the thoughts that had been bothering her.

The doctor looked annoyed and reacted. "This has got nothing to do with the hospital. Such patients are always hanging by a thin thread of life…even a small thing can magnify their suffering."

This sounded like an extreme descriptor for a person who had been able to function on his own until three weeks back, albeit a lot slower than he would like.

Ninjja's sister, who had been quiet so far, cleared her throat and asked a point-blank question: "Are you saying that he is living on borrowed time? What is the typical life expectancy of patients in stage-four COPD?"

Ninjja was surprised by her directness. A near-death experience had transformed her from an overemotional person to someone who could talk about death in a dispassionate way.

"Such patients have to be watched from winter to winter. The life expectancy could be anywhere from one year to ten years," the doctor responded after resuming his cool. He then went on to describe a case history of someone who was in much worse shape than her dad and then went on to live for ten years.

Ninjja wasn't sure if she was supposed to become depressed or find solace with this information. She was sitting face-to-face with another character, "SuperMeDoc" who considered his specialist tag to mean that his views were supreme and there wasn't any possibility of a debate.

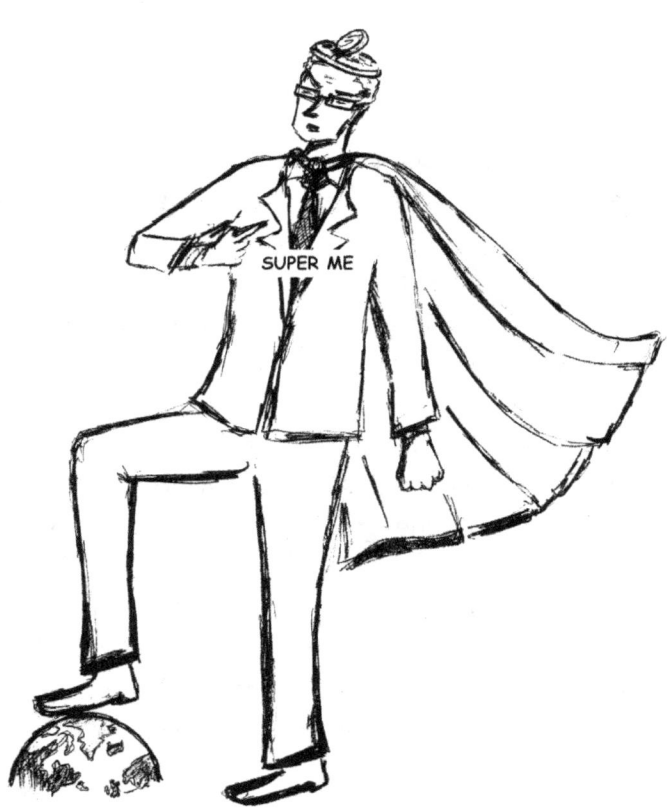

As there was nothing more to do, the sisters took some guidance on lifestyle management and things to watch out for before heading out with heavy hearts.

"There is something that still doesn't fit," Ninjja said to her sister once they were in the car. "If our father is indeed in such an advanced stage of COPD, an experienced specialist should have been able to diagnose it just by looking at the patient and seeing his X-ray and CT scans. Why didn't he mention the diagnosis of COPD before performing the bronchoscopy?"

"Yeah, you are right…I have been reading about this doctor on the internet, and he is clearly one of the few top-notch doctors in this field. Clearly this cannot be attributed to a lack of expertise or experience." Her sister was on the same track with her now.

"One can understand the need for a bronchoscopy to rule out the possibility of cancer, but it is difficult to imagine that the doctor could not diagnose the presence of COPD before seeing the fluttering windpipe through the bronchoscope…"

She was interrupted by the guard at the main gate to collect the parking charges.

"Let's speak to the doctor who was treating him earlier in our hometown," Ninjja added thoughtfully, and she handed over her cell phone. Ninjja's sister took the lead and briefed the doctor about new developments. There was a surprise awaiting them.

"Yes, he was suffering from COPD even here. What's new?" the doctor responded coolly.

The sisters were taken aback. "But the patient does not know about this...even his prescription doesn't mention this disease." Ninjja was now becoming numb with frustration. The doctor was unfazed and did not think he had committed any folly by keeping the patient in the dark. He replied with the same composure, "I am very clear; I was treating him for COPD."

"Based on the prescriptions, we always thought he was suffering from asthma and bronchitis. Had we known about this lethal disease, we could have managed his lifestyle much more wisely." Ninjja's sister made one last attempt at highlighting the value of transparency in treatment. There was no point in digging up old graves, however, so they finally thanked the doctor and ended the call on a cordial note.

"Wow, this is amazing. In the United States, they tell you lot more than you would want to know and can handle; here we are at the other extreme. Either they believe that the patient is a complete idiot, or they are overprotective lest the patient should panic." Ninjja's sister was still in a mode of disbelief. "Had we known how this disease progresses, we could have been more regimented about physiotherapy; we could have started oxygen therapy much sooner; mild steroids could have been started...our father wouldn't have had to suffer so much." Ninjja's sister ended her dialogue with a tinge of high emotion.

But Ninjja was on a different plane. She started off on the point that had been bugging her for so long: "Looks like it was not that difficult to diagnose COPD after all...in that case, why didn't the doctors in this reputed big-city hospital first try to stabilize his situation with steroids and all the other things that they did later before proceeding to do a bronchoscopy?" Ninjja could feel the pain growing inside her.

The car had reached its destination. Ninjja did not want her mother to get worked up over this turmoil, so she appropriately sealed the lid and asked her sister to do the same. They walked in with forced smiles that were too easy to detect. However, their mother decided to let them be happy with their deceit and proceeded to behave normally. It was bizarre. They were all pretending to be normal and hiding their true emotions in the false hope that the others would feel better this way.

Their father looked restful in his sleep, though Ninjja knew that it was a farce. He was physically and emotionally so shaken up that taking him to any other doctor was next to impossible. Given the modern evolution of health-care in big cities, no doctor was willing to pay a home visit. The only consistent answer that she got was to bring him back to the hospital and admit him for a few days. Ninjja had never felt so helpless before in her life. It was time to tap into her friends' network with a desperate cry for help.

After a couple of days, two leads emerged. One was through a friend of Arv's, and another was through an office colleague. Ninjja and her sister prepared the case history with great diligence and were ready to rattle out the summary even in their sleep. They had to be on top of all the details to make up for the patient's absence.

A good hour and a half separated them from the hospital they were visiting to get another perspective. The same ever-expanding metros that acted as a magnet for medical talent across the country acted as a barrier between them and the patients through sheer congestion. Ninjja could not imagine how her father would have survived this journey through cratered roads and the incessant honking necessary to survive in wild traffic.

After the regular procedures at the hospital, they were finally seated outside the doctor's office. The doctor received them with eye contact and a smile that positively surprised Ninjja. Perhaps the personal reference deserved to be thanked for this welcoming approach.

The doctor was pleased to see the well-organized case history and the structured narration that accompanied it. He confirmed the line of treatment, with some minor tweaks to take care of the adverse effects attributable to steroids. Ninjja set aside some of the other issues that she wanted to discuss and moved to the difficult question that had been bothering her for several weeks: "Doctor, where do you see the lump in this X-ray and the CT scan?"

She got the reply that she had been dreading: "There is no lump that can be seen here." He had pulled up the CT scan on his computer screen and went on to explain very patiently, "What you see here are air pockets, and they indicate an advanced stage of COPD."

"In that case, the bronchoscopy was not needed," Ninjja blurted out instantly, feeling a deep sense of anguish. "Do you think my father's health could have destabilized because of this procedure?"

The doctor realized the direction she was heading in and maintained the official line: "The procedure is supposed to be harmless; it can't be expected to make the situation worse. It may have just helped in confirming the actual position." Ninjja was cognizant of the fact that it would be difficult to directly negate the judgment of a senior individual from the same profession. However harmless the procedure was, Arv's words regarding the concept of equilibrium were coming back to haunt her.

She was thankful that the doctor did not hide his own judgment on the reports. He happily answered all the follow-up questions, and upon Ninjja's request, he offered to send one of his interns for a home visit to check and give the doctor the needed feedback. Ninjja and her sister felt indebted to his gesture and could not thank him enough.

On their way back, Ninjja started off: "I can't believe that I am so dumb. Why did I believe them when they said there was a lump? Why didn't I question their interpretation? I should have paused before giving the green light for an invasive test...all of this is my fault." Ninjja's tone was full of remorse and guilt.

"Stop blaming yourself. You can't be held guilty for trusting the judgment of two doctors, including a specialist of a reputed hospital! After someone scares you about the possibility of cancer, I don't think any normal human being would like to delay the test that is required to prove or disprove it."

"But why didn't I read the signs? There was a delay in getting the X-ray report; then I was out of town, which should have been taken as a reason to delay the test...the doctor that I spoke to through a friend had mentioned that it is hard to tell without seeing the report...However, I went by the latter half of his statement that the test is harmless." Ninjja's anguish was not letting her stop.

"Stop behaving like a superstitious thickhead! Try to remember the stress that you were under when the decision was taken. The doctors had scared our mother enough that she wanted to get to the truth as soon as possible. You were told that it was not wise to delay the test. Either you would have needed to be a superhuman or a doctor yourself to go against the recommendation in this case."

Ninjja calmed down a little, but she could now see the critical angle that she had missed earlier. As both of the doctors came from the same hospital, the possibility of bias could not be ruled out. Beyond financial gain (which, of course, came in the form of the extended stay at the hospital), the test also contributed to the overall statistics of the hospital as well as of the specialist.

During her readings later about the specialists in this field, Ninjja realized that the number of bronchoscopies performed was one of the parameters mentioned in establishing doctors' reputations. "Do you think our dad was being used just as a statistics booster or as a guinea pig for training new doctors?" Ninjja spoke with the angst of someone who is stung by the guardian angel himself.

Ninjja's sister could not rebuke her anymore, as the statement was piercing enough to cause her equal or more pain. While what was needed was a vehement dismissal of Ninjja's question to save her from increasing agony, Ninjja's sister could muster only a weak plea to let bygones be bygones.

She signed off with her gaze fixed at some unknown point outside the window. Ninjja followed her gaze and wondered if her sister was hoping to dissolve the wrong into infinity and undo the damage done.

Ninjja went to bed with a heavy heart that night. She wanted to believe that there was an error in judgment of the doctors, but there were more compelling arguments to suspect willful wrongdoing. Even though the outcome of both the follies was the same, she wasn't sure what would be more hurtful: a lacuna on the skill dimension or on the dimension of will. Unfortunately, suing the hospital or the doctor was not something that the common man can think of in India.

To forget and forgive is the only option available to a peace-loving person in a country where, even in cases of blatant crimes, the chances of timely justice are no better than a draw of roulette. Ninjja tried to take the high road, as preached by the wise men, and hoped that killing part of her memory would help her find peace with herself.

The visit to the second specialist was helpful yet agonizing. He used a more polite and politically correct expression to describe what had happened: "There is only a very weak indication for the need for a bronchoscopy," he commented without removing his eyes from the multitude of test reports sitting on his desk.

Ninjja controlled her anguish and directed a forward-looking question at him: "I have seen several mentions of physiotherapy for COPD. Does it really help?"

"Yes, of course...physiotherapy can yield phenomenal results if done properly and regularly."

"Is there someone you can recommend to do the sessions at home?" Ninjja's sister was eager to get to some concrete solutions.

"Sorry, I won't be able to help you there. I don't know anyone who provides home-based physiotherapy," the doctor replied with some hesitation. Ninjja was surprised. One would have expected a leading hospital to be able to offer a solution spanning different therapies, and the lead doctor seemed like the logical candidate to be able to offer the integrated solution, let alone just help with the navigation!

The doctor saw the mixed feelings of surprise and confusion written all over their faces and tried to mend the situation. "The senior doctor from neurology who referred you to me is very well connected. If he talks to the physiotherapy department, something might be worked out." He hoped that there would be no further questions.

Ninjja knew that, despite falling short of the need of the hour by miles, the doctor was doing whatever he could do within his limits. She chose to follow his lead and dived back into the "white wall" of nurses and attendants on the floor above. As expected, meeting the doctor was not easy. The mythical guards of heaven stood between them and the doctor, and the only available door was through the billing desk.

The senior doctor was very kind and gave them a patient hearing. He noticed the billing document that Ninjja had inadvertently kept on the table along with other documents and was visibly upset. "Well, you haven't come to a neurosurgeon for his advice on a respiratory disorder...this billing for my consultation isn't fair..." he mumbled and he scribbled "Please refund" on the bill in a jiffy. He sprang into action immediately; with a couple of phone calls, the home support of a physiotherapist was arranged. He reassured them that he would be available to help them anytime they needed. Ninjja and her sister were touched by his caring gesture, which was quite unlike the transactional world that he was operating in.

"What if we didn't come here through a personal connection? We would have been lost in the system," Ninjja's sister remarked. The lack of a system that provided equal opportunities and transparency to each person who came to the hospital continued to irritate Ninjja like a thorn stuck in her heel.

The young physiotherapist who showed up that evening did not inspire much confidence with his inexperienced look, but his tremendous patience in dealing with a patient who had given up on life was enough to make Ninjja grant him the opportunity for a fair try.

In addition, every piece of knowledge that they could find on alternative therapies in the form of foods to take, foods to avoid, and natural energy supplements were put into practice with a zeal as though there were no tomorrow. This was war on COPD! The scale of operations had become overwhelming for Ninjja's mother. Ninjja promptly prepared an hourly chart with a listing of medicines, therapies, food, and so forth on a large A3 sheet and professionally displayed it on a pinup board. To enable tracking, Ninjja also provided removable, sticky red dots to mark the tasks that were completed for the day.

Apart from providing some unexpected giggles to all the visitors who came in with grim looks on their faces, this professionally done sheet of paper did serve some useful purpose—it made the colossal task actually doable! Ninjja couldn't comprehend what was so funny about using techniques that were used to manage and track complex projects in professional companies, but she wasn't complaining about the side benefit that her handiwork was providing.

A heavy-duty combination of medicinal and nutritional interventions, along with the physiotherapist's hard work, put Ninjja's dad back on his feet.

After ten days, when he finally climbed down a flight of stairs and walked in the park without any support, the excitement it offered to the family was equivalent to the time when Ninjja's little niece had taken her first baby steps before falling back onto the floor.

This small preview suggested that life might be back on track again for her dad. Hopefully, even the second folly by the doctor of too-quick a reduction in steroid dosage (in addition to the first one, the wrong diagnosis regarding the lump) was now somewhat negated and had offered a third lease of life to her father. This dreadful conjecture regarding two consecutive errors by doctors was now confirmed through interactions with other specialists as well and had accentuated Ninjja's self-inflicted feeling of guilt.

While Ninjja was trying to cope with the ghosts that were haunting her, she felt that the gaping holes in the service of the hospitals were equally intimidating.

Taking on an optimistic lens, even if one were to take the fortunate scenario of no intentional errors by the hospital, there was absolutely no consideration in the hospital's operating procedures for the trauma that the family experienced. The fact that stress affected people's thinking and decision-making ability should not be an unknown fact to those in the business of treating people.

To top it all, the one-way flow of information, delivered in a hurried manner, could hardly be considered helpful for the harried family members. Could they be expected to make the right choices under such a backdrop?

As Ninjja thought more broadly about different critical situations, she was surprised to see that the list of potential choices during the hospital stay and after discharge was not a short one. For example:

- There may be a choice to have surgery or other invasive procedures or to opt for a longer treatment that may not lessen the immediate pain. Going for alternative therapies or stopping treatment altogether might be a realistic choice as well. It is possible that the consulting doctor presents only a narrow range of choices to begin with!
- Continue the hospital stay or opt for home care?
- Postdischarge follow-ups with the general physician or go to one of the specialists who attended to the patient during the hospital stay?
- Put in effort and money now on supporting therapies vs. face the probable implications later in life? In some cases, ignoring supporting therapies might be fine in the short term, but can create debilitating effects many years down the line.

The fact that most people went through the ordeal without even knowing that there were choices or exercised their decision-making powers with sketchy information was scary enough for Ninjja. *Clearly there is a need to help the family members (and the patient) with their emotional state and engage in a discussion of the pros and cons of different choices.*

The practical challenges of getting the busy critical-care doctors to spend time with patients was not lost on Ninjja. This challenge was similar in some ways to what Ninjja had encountered with her corporate clients. Often the line managers were so caught up with day-to-day firefighting that there was no time to step back, think, and engage in the big picture. This gap gave birth to consulting services and internal think tanks.

While the role of such groups was crucial for the long-term survival of an organization, in the current context of health-care, it was necessary only for the well-being of the patient (and not necessarily the health-care provider).

While the corporations found it worth their money to invest in such resources, the hospitals might find themselves losing short-term revenue opportunities through improving the knowledge of their patients! Though there was a clear need, Ninjja struggled to find the motivation until she expanded her horizons.

Over the longer term, one needs to believe that resultant metrics like lower error rates, faster recovery of patients, and better customer satisfaction would be of interest to the hospitals as well. *If only there were such a long-term perspective!* Ninjja sighed. Given the sensitive nature of this support, ideally, this should be free for critical-care patients. However, creating an independent value proposition centered on this unmet need of customers was certainly a possibility. Ninjja hoped that some social entrepreneurs would find the idea valuable enough to set up a business around it. The success of any such service would depend on the choice of the right counselors, though—that is, doctors with a holistic perspective, the right mind-set, and empathy (and not necessarily seniority).

• • •

Ninjja's thought process was interrupted by a feeble voice in the background. As she turned back, she was pleasantly surprised to see her dad calling out for her.

He had managed to get up from the bed on his own, had found his balance with the support of a stick, and had walked across ten steps to proudly announce his stupendous progress. Ninjja was moved to see this display of enthusiasm and positivity toward life. She instantly reciprocated with a bright smile and tried to seat him comfortably in his favorite chair. Ninjja was really proud of her dad, who was happily celebrating these miniscule successes instead of brooding over several things that had horribly gone wrong (often because of gross callousness) in the past month. He had barely settled in when a visitor dropped by to meet him.

Ninjja's father gave him the best possible welcome that was feasible in his current state.

"Meet my latest friend, who will be here with me for the rest of my life," he said jovially, referring to the oxygen machine that was parked next to his chair. It was ironic that everyone was smiling in such a grim situation. Ninjja silently saluted her father's joie de vivre and hoped that at least a small fraction of this trait had been genetically transferred to her.

Ten

The New Equilibrium

FEBRUARY 2011

Everyone had returned to their respective normal lives, except for Ninjja's father and mother. Her dad was doing well; that is, he was able to function without the external oxygen support for three to four hours at a time. However, there was a big routine of medications, therapies, exercises, and food intake that had become a fulcrum around which Ninjja's mother had started revolving.

Ninjja's sister was back in the United States and was trying to do her best from far away. She would religiously call twice a day to provide emotional support and did whatever she could using the Internet, like finding more information and searching for home-care agencies, and she had managed to get a twelve-hour attendant to ease her mother's burden—at a hefty price.

However, this critical service didn't come without the typical labor-related problems that every Indian industry encountered. Absenteeism, reporting late for work, not following the instructions properly, and having a new person every few days who had to be instructed from scratch was part and parcel of the service. Given that having some support was better than having no support at all, the family continued to put up with this daylight fleecing in the name of home-care support.

As far as Ninjja was concerned, she was left standing holding the bag for all the sundry to-dos and emergency support.

After going through the ordeal of the past several months, Ninjja's mother had grown so panicky that Ninjja's number had become the "911" that could be dialed 24-7 for the slightest sneeze that didn't feel normal.

Ninjja was glad that her colleagues were sensitive enough to put up with her if she excused herself in the middle of an important meeting to take a call. These urgent calls that came her way varied from zero to ten on the criticality scale, but there was no way for Ninjja to help her mother recalibrate.

Ninjja's father was so full of enthusiasm that he wanted to really live those few hours where he did not have to stay chained to the oxygen machine. He would use that time to walk up to the little market within the housing complex or hop across to a neighbor's home. To avoid the strict controls on his long list of dos and don'ts, Ninjja's dad had started indulging in his old habit of not informing her mother regarding his route plan or the duration for which he was planning to stay outside.

The attendant had become his silent accomplice, which had the effect of adding a handful of salt to Ninjja's mother's already hypertensive persona.

While Ninjja could understand her mother's agony, the cuteness of her dad's mischievous behavior really prevented her from taking any sides.

Having observed his progress over the past few weeks, Ninjja felt that he was now fit enough for a small outing and hoped that it would help satiate his need for being out in the open. Ninjja's mother had become so overcautious that she became extremely jittery at even the thought of taking him out to a mall for few hours. Ninjja was faced with a barrage of questions—"What if he gets breathless? What if he gets very tired? What if there is dust?"

Unfortunately, there were not many options left for an outing, if one had to find a place that did not have dust in a city that was in a state of perpetual construction. Using a combination of reasoning and bullying techniques, Ninjja finally got her mother to agree to her proposition.

Ninjja offered to carry an oxygen cylinder in the car as a backup, a wheelchair in the trunk, and the emergency inhaler for a sudden attack; and she promised to be within fifteen minutes of driving distance of their home. Doing anything beyond this wasn't possible even with any other arsenal.

Ninjja's dad was so excited at the thought of being able to step out of his situation of house arrest that he spent most of the evening planning for the outing the next day. His joy was no less than what his three-year-old granddaughter felt at being allowed to play in dirt and mud in the park after recovering from a bout of sickness.

When Ninjja arrived to pick up her parents, she was elated to see her dad dressed in his most favorite kurta (a long shirt) and khadi (an Indian homespun cotton cloth) jacket. He was holding his stylish walking stick and was all set to go. The attendant looked excited to get a break from his regular drudgery. The only person who couldn't rejoice in the moment was Ninjja's mother, as the fear of the unknown was biting her.

The trip went very well. The wheelchair came in handy during the long walk from the parking lot to the mall, and fortunately, they did not need to use any other items in their arsenal. The activities that they indulged in at the mall would otherwise pass off as very dull and uninspiring (to be precise, they ended up buying groceries and having a cup of coffee); but the context for this event made it totally memorable. Being in a lively place rejuvenated Ninjja's dad so much that he ended up walking back to the car instead of riding in his wheelchair.

• • •

The next morning, Ninjja's father woke up with a high fever. The hide-and-seek between joy and sorrow was far from over.

Ninjja was back on her guilt trip when her dad intervened: "The fever could have caught me anywhere if it had to—going to the mall has got nothing to do with it. So, just stop thinking about it. It will go away."

Ninjja knew in her heart that any infection in his condition had the potential of turning fatal, but she kept her thoughts to herself and tried to maintain a positive face. A few days and several antibiotics later, her father was on the path of recovery again.

It wasn't until their second trip to the mall, a month later, that she realized that spending time at any enclosed public place was indeed a source of risk for her father in his newly acquired delicate condition. Ninjja asked the doctor directly about her theory and, sadly, had it confirmed.

While curiosity drives one to confirm one's worst fears, it is ironic that knowledge of the truth at times makes life even more difficult.

Ninjja didn't know whether this new discovery was a cause to rejoice, as they now knew one more critical trick to avoid infections, or if it was a reason enough to be saddened, as there were now more shackles imposed on her father's already constrained living. It was a scary thought that each and every move, each and every breath that her dad took, had to be well-thought-out.

What he was expected to do now was in such a sharp contrast to his natural, gregarious self that Ninjja was tempted to conceal this information. "Let him live to his fullest for whatever time God has given him...why should I spoil his small pleasures and take away the joy of living?" she said to herself with an unsure feeling.

A few days later, as Ninjja turned around to park her car, she saw her dad happily chatting away with someone who had a severe cough and cold. She hurriedly got out of the car and instinctively found herself coaxing her dad to go back upstairs. It felt like her defense mechanism had kicked in unknowingly, with all her faculties focused on curtailing her dad's exposure to another potential threat! Ninjja already knew that certain weather conditions were a critical testing time for her father's health. The newly discovered additional burden of risk due to human exposure was now overwhelming her.

Is it even possible to design a life that is so isolated from human interaction and the very environment that one is born in?

In her moment of deep despair, Ninjja dialed Arv's number. There was no response.

Instinctively, she moved on to dial Uma.

"Hello! Think of the devil and..." Uma said in a peppy tone.

Unlike in all their other, normal calls, Uma dramatically reduced her share of words and listened patiently. She empathized with Ninjja, complying with the need of the hour. It helped Ninjja calm down and got her into a receptive mind frame.

"Tell me, what should I do?" Ninjja was eagerly looking for clear answers.

"Your concern and love for your father is forcing you to make decisions on his behalf that you believe would be good for him...am I right?" asked Uma.

"What do you expect me to do? Scaring him about everything around him would be like condemning him to a miserable life," Ninjja said anxiously.

"Do you think you will be able to protect him if he doesn't even know what could hurt him? Will you be there with him all the time to usher him away from someone who is sneezing or suffering from viral infection?"

"What if I just let him be his natural self and face the consequences as God's will? Maybe nothing will happen!" Ninjja said, hoping against hope.

Uma now adopted her typical motherly tone. "No, you can't do that! You can't deprive your dad of vital information that has a bearing on how he leads his life! If he were mentally unfit, I could understand your rationale, but not under the current circumstances." She paused to see if her authoritative approach had moved the dial even a bit in Ninjja's head.

For once, Ninjja was glad that Uma was not a consultant. Uma did not present her with three options that had elaborate details of pros and cons but instead put forward a firm view. It was this conviction that was the need of the hour.

This was a time when Ninjja's head was so cluttered that her mental prowess to sift through the pros and cons to make a final call was severely limited. Ninjja thanked Uma for not testing her ability to do mental acrobatics and for clearly speaking her mind.

"But how will I talk to Mother? She is so hyper about everything… how do you think this will play out? She might just pass a restraining order to limit anyone coming within few hundred meters of my dad," Ninjja blurted out, voicing her worst fears.

Uma continued, keeping the upper hand in the conversation. "You will need to try. I can try to help as well. I have a good rapport with your mother…maybe she will pay more attention to me as an outsider. What say you?" Ninjja was silent. "Hey…you are not thinking about maintaining the status quo…are you?" Uma tried to nudge the silence on the other end of phone.

"Mmm…no…no, I was just thinking…" Ninjja mumbled with the guilt of someone who was caught red-handed.

Finally, it was time to hit the end button on the phone, and they parted with an agreement to discuss Ninjja's progress the next day.

. . .

The next few days were difficult as Ninjja went about disseminating smaller packets of bad news instead of a bumper dosage. Her father was going through a range of emotions—from despair to fear to indifference. The slow motion made sure that the implications were somewhat understood, at least. Ninjja was glad that she had prolonged her own agony over several days to ease the pain of this discovery for her parents.

"Father, there are young children who suffer from even more scary conditions, and the worst part is, they can't even be expected to watch out for some of the dangers. Have you heard of nut allergies? Or hemophilia, when even a small cut on the body can prove lethal? Even these children don't isolate themselves from the world. They go to a regular school, play with other kids, and have some special assistance to take care of emergencies.

"So the bottom line is, you are not going to be under house arrest! The only principle that you have to follow is to keep your eyes and ears open. If you see an open pit, please don't jump into it! For example, if you can see a person with a red nose and watery eyes, there is no need to indulge in polite conversation. You can always make a quick exit. Do you understand?" Ninjja paused to see if her practical advice had made any impression on her father.

He nodded like a small child who was thoroughly bored with all the preaching thrust on him. Ninjja took this as a signal to put a stopper in her mouth. It was easier to preach to her parents that there was no need to worry than to actually internalize it herself. Ninjja decided to leave the future to the hopeless person's last defense—destiny!

• • •

APRIL 2011

Winter was formally over, and the summer hadn't reached its youth. It was one of the few pleasant days that one was graced with in Delhi.

Work was going on at a very hectic pace. During this period, Ninjja's father's enthusiasm was inversely proportional to the time that she had on hand. If she forgot to call her father in the morning or couldn't meet him, his acute need for affection would force him to call her multiple times. Ninjja was finding it difficult to cope with conflicting demands.

"Father, I am in the middle of a critical meeting. Is there anything urgent?" Ninjja answered her phone in an irritated tone.

Her father was in a bright mood and replied, unperturbed by her response, "Nothing, my child; I was missing you. Will I be seeing you this evening?"

"I am not sure. I might get in very late. I will talk to you later," Ninjja said quickly and hung up.

She apologized to her colleagues and resumed the meeting. A part of her brain was still going over her abrupt response and making her a tad uncomfortable. The day slipped by, and Ninjja didn't get any time to call her dad back. By the time she reached home, he was fast asleep. Needless to say, it did not help her uncomfortable feeling one bit.

Ninjja was in bed, but her mind couldn't find the peace that was necessary to get good sleep. At some level, she felt that her father was now more like a child who needed constant love and attention, and yet he was old enough that one couldn't admonish him for his childlike behavior. Ninjja started wondering if her situation was better or worse than that of a mother who was unable to give the time demanded by her child. With every passing day, a child becomes stronger and shows hope for a brighter tomorrow. In her own situation, Ninjja didn't know what tomorrow would be like. There was no such hope that her father would regain all his lost strength. The time that he had remaining was unknown, and every passing day was reducing the time that he had with his loved ones. Whatever there was—it was the current moment! Ninjja wanted to make sure that her dad remained happy and lived that moment to the fullest. And yet, she was failing… he wanted to have her around for more than she could manage…

Ninjja had a curtain of tears that night between her and her dreams.

· · ·

Two days later, Arv invited her to have coffee to celebrate the fact that his office had moved to the building next to Ninjja's. Ten minutes into the conversation, he changed the subject. "Is something on your mind?" he asked.

That was the perfect opening to get Ninjja to pour out her emotions. Arv was sipping his black coffee at a leisurely pace, giving Ninjja ample time to share her feelings. Finally, she stopped and glanced at her lukewarm coffee, which bore testimony to her monologue as well as to Arv's patience.

"Well, I hear you. I have no experience in this regard, but whatever you are feeling seems normal to me. You are trying to accomplish something that would need two of you—how can you be in two places at the same time? Even if we take a scenario where you take some time off, the question is, for how long? Will it be a month...six months...five years, ten years? What happens to your own life, your aspirations, in the meanwhile? Whenever you resume work, the same dilemma will continue. And by the way, if you stay out of work for too long, there may not be any work left for you later." Arv paused.

"Are you suggesting that I act selfishly and dump my father? How will I ever be able to live with myself in that case?"

Arv was in no mood to interject.

Ninjja paused for few moments and then continued, "Or maybe I need to start setting some realistic expectations for myself. I can't be a superhuman, after all."

Arv was glad that Ninjja was trying to discover the answer for herself.

True to everything else in life, there wasn't a perfect answer. There were trade-offs to be made! Ninjja decided to have a one more go at explaining the pressures of the modern-day working environment to her father. She also reminded herself to be a lot more patient. How could she even imagine that her father, a former professor of literature would communicate to her in bullet points? There were no shortcuts to the elaborate story-telling style that her father loved to communicate in. It was ironic that the same trait that had regaled her during her growing-up days had turned into a challenge due to the paucity of time.

Ninjja realized that she had received counseling unknowingly without having to go to a therapist. She was thankful that she had such phenomenal support from friends that helped her with maintaining sanity.

"Having close friends is like having a comfortable home in bad weather that is never valued! One takes it as a given. The real value is not understood till one is deprived of it," Ninjja wrote in her diary that night.

• • •

JULY 2011

While the early showers of monsoon season had brought pleasure to the most sun-scorched citizens, the dark clouds had the reverse impact on her father—they plunged him into depression. Soon he started experiencing breathing difficulty. Apparently the two phenomena were linked, but there were different theories as to which came first.

The attending specialist who had initially triggered the downslide and then later resurrected her dad was away. Ninjja thought this might be an opportunity to consult another doctor.

While Ninjja definitely believed that the invasive test procedure was the key driver of the steep deterioration in her father's condition, her parents were from the "doctor is God" era and continued to believe that the doctor had made all the right decisions for them. Over time, Ninjja's father had also developed a personal rapport with the doctor that was beyond the normal doctor-patient relationship.

There was a comfort zone that often translated to a standard excuse for not visiting anyone else.

The doctor's recommendation of increasing steroids was further aggravating her father's depression, sapping him of his energy and desire to step out of the home.

Three days later, having patiently listened to the long list of complaints that were magnified by her father's depressive state, the doctor concluded that it was time to end the long-distance advisory and suggested that Ninjja's father visit the hospital and meet one of his juniors.

After several hours of confusion, the decision was made to visit the alternate specialist instead of the junior doctor. Ninjja still had the option to call the new specialist and request for some latitude, thanks to the personal reference that she had. Ninjja decided to use that chip.

"Doctor, I am...umm...do you remember me? I came through the reference of..." Ninjja started off. After getting a sense of recall at the other end, she continued, "I have a request. I want to bring my father for your consultation...but he is feeling very weak. I don't think he will be able to sit around for long in the waiting area. Could you please suggest a time when you will be able to see him quickly?" Ninjja's tone was genuine.

The doctor obliged. "Sure. Why don't you come to the emergency area during the regular visiting hours? Give me a call once you arrive. It will be much easier for me to skip any queues that way, and your father will also be more comfortable there."

That did sound like a plan.

• • •

Ninjja took the next day off and braced herself for the task ahead. Getting a depressed, weak, old man into a car for a fifteen-minute drive to the hospital was easier said than done. It took over an hour of counseling and cajoling to get the desired movement.

Seeing her father go through such mood swings from full exuberance to total despair, in addition to his physical problem, was killing her. She had read that mental strength was key to managing and surviving COPD. Sadly, this was not going to be one of the strengths that they could rely on.

Once at the emergency entrance, Ninjja called the doctor and asked him to come down at his earliest convenience. The hospital attendants were efficient enough to bring a wheelchair quickly and helped her father disembark. Ninjja's mother accompanied her father inside, while Ninjja proceeded to the gigantic parking lot in the basement.

The process of getting a parking ticket, finding a spot, parking, and then walking back to the emergency area ended up consuming fifteen minutes despite efficiency at each step.

Ninjja was surprised when she did not see her parents outside the emergency area. Upon enquiry, she was informed that her father was inside the emergency room. The sight that was awaiting her was nothing short of a shocker:

Ninjja's father was lying on the hospital bed with several apparatuses attached to his body, and there were at least five people hovering around him. Ninjja's mother was standing next to the bed in a state of complete shock. She was trying to explain to the attending staff that they could use the oxygen cylinder that Ninjja's father was already using, but no one bothered to listen. Ninjja's father was looking totally ruffled and nervous. He had almost lost his voice.

Ninjja failed to understand how the medical staff had succeeded in unleashing such a panic within fifteen minutes!

After the first minute of shock, the next emotion that overpowered Ninjja was anger. "What's going on here? We are waiting here to consult Dr. Gupta. Why have you all started treating my father?" Ninjja shouted. None of the hospital staff was interested in giving her a reply.

Ninjja's mother meekly murmured, "I tried telling them the same thing…but they said he was in a bad shape and needed immediate attention."

This infuriated Ninjja further. "Can someone please explain? Where is Dr. Gupta?" she screamed again.

This time around, one of the nurses turned to her and said, "The emergency in charge is Dr. Sharma; we are acting under his instructions."

Without wasting any more time, Ninjja called up the specialist again. "Doctor Gupta, I have no idea what's happening here. We have come for a consultation, and the folks down here have already started some treatment. Could you please instruct them to stop and wait for you? How long will you take?"

"Oh, don't worry. I will speak to the emergency room. I have already sent my assistant doctor. I will be there with you as soon as I can," he said in a reassuring tone. Ninjja decided to not to pressure him further, mindful of the stresses that the doctors had to operate under.

Ninjja had barely deposited the phone back in her purse when she noticed that the saga was still continuing. A needle had already been pricked into her father's arm. "No injections, please. Just stop whatever you are doing," Ninjja screamed again.

"We are just taking a blood sample," came the calm reply. Before Ninjja could comprehend the need for all these tests, two more people came in hurriedly and thrust a portable machine in front of her father's chest.

"Now what's this?" Ninjja questioned again.

"We have to take a chest X-ray." An X-ray, given his lung situation, did not seem illogical, so Ninjja refrained from protesting again. However, she noticed that her father was saying something that no one was bothering to pay attention to. She stepped closer to him and asked him to repeat whatever his concern was. To her surprise, her father was saying that the X-ray had already been taken. "When did they take the X-ray, Father?" she asked slowly to confirm if she had heard him correctly.

"When you were away…" he replied slowly.

Ninjja's mother was so flabbergasted with all the action that she had only some confused memory of the events that were going on. It seemed unlikely that within the first fifteen minutes, the hospital staff would have been swift enough to get a portable X-ray machine and execute the job. Was it her father's weak physical and mental state that was leading to this confusion? However, Ninjja decided to believe that her father's supersharp brain still had some firepower left, and whatever he was saying was true. "Please stop," Ninjja said in a stern voice, startling the two new actors in this drama. "Can you please pay attention to what the patient has to say? He says that the X-ray has been taken already." Her voice was so stern now that they could not afford to ignore it.

"Look, we have been instructed to take the X-ray," they tried to explain, pointing her to a piece of paper in their hands.

"I am not doubting that. I am just saying that it has probably been taken. I am sure you don't want the patient doubly exposed to X-rays. Can you please cross-check?" Ninjja tried to soften her tone.

Fortunately, they found it befitting to accede to Ninjja's request and scurried away to reconfirm the status. Soon after, to their shock, they realized that Ninjja's father was right.

The attendants had barely left the bedside when a busy-looking young lady arrived on the scene. She quickly glanced at the monitors and started rattling out numerous tests that she wanted done. The nurse was scampering to keep up with her speed. Ninjja guessed that she might be the assistant doctor that the senior doctor was referring to. Ninjja found it a bit odd that the new doctor didn't even bother talking to the patient's family before getting into the instruction phase.

While Ninjja was debating if she should go forward and speak to the doctor, she overheard something that alarmed her. "And please give him a hydrocortisone injection right away."

Ninjja's instant reaction was to jump in with a big bang. "Are you suggesting an injection? Did you say hydrocortisone?"

The doctor was startled and finally noticed the harried family standing next to the patient. "Yes," she replied. "Are you a doctor as well?"

Ninjja told her that she had been discussing various options of treatment with doctors over the past several months and had heard about the injection. "As far as I am aware, a few days of hospital stay becomes necessary after this injection. Also, my understanding is that the patient gets used to this injection and has to be brought back to the hospital more often." Ninjja tried to appear confident while making this assertion.

The lady in question was unmoved and answered with a straight face, "The patient is in bad shape, so this is needed." She continued with the instructions regarding the injection with a sense of purpose. She had no inclination to even make eye contact, lest she get caught up in talking to the patient or his family. Ninjja felt an uncontrollable panic brewing inside her, forcing her into pleading mode. "Please, can you wait just for a few minutes? I can't have any medication administered till I speak to Dr. Gupta. He is aware of my father's history, and I would like him to have a look first... please...hope you understand." Ninjja paused, anticipating a favorable response.

The young lady threw up her hands in frustration and walked away without saying another word. Ninjja had potentially hurt the young doctor's sense of control, power, and enthusiasm.

Given what was at stake, Ninjja felt no sense of remorse at her own behavior. The caricature of this doctor, who she named as "DocNoIcontact" was bemusing and annoying at the same time.

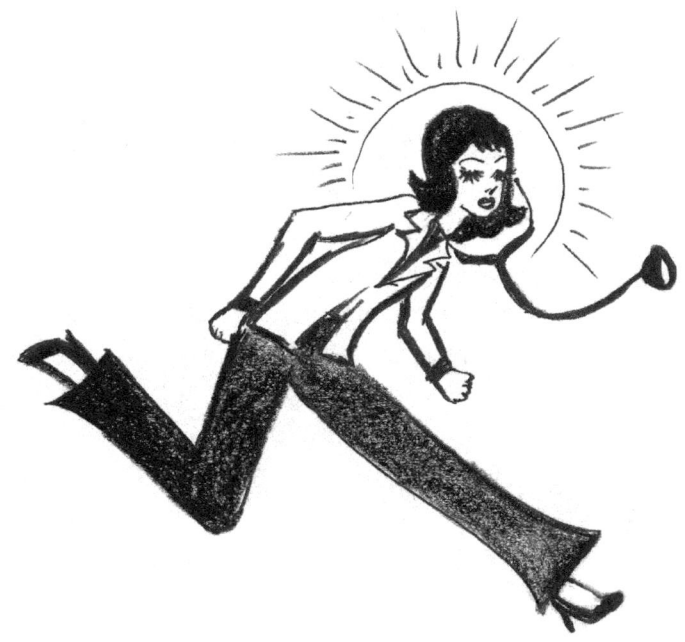

DocNoIcontact: Extremely busy; has no time to converse with patients. Has a master list of all the tests that is dished out before anyone has a chance to blink an eye!

Ten minutes later, the attending crowd had petered out for want of any opportunity for meaningful action on the patient. Ninjja was guilty of decimating their exciting job content. Finally, Dr. Gupta arrived on the scene. He apologized for the delay and proceeded to talk to the patient and his family (apart from looking at the plethora of statistics that had been put on display).

"He doesn't look very good. It will be good to keep him under observation. We may need to use the injection to stabilize the situation," he commented. While the advice regarding observation made sense, by now Ninjja was wise enough to know that the real observers would be attendants and junior doctors, with a fleeting visit from the senior doctor. The bigger challenge that scared her was that the observers were never satisfied with observation alone; they were itching for action! It was a common human psychology. If one were to go back home and tell a story about the day's work, how dull and boring would it be to say, "I talked to the patient and gave couple of medicines to help him feel better." The more action-filled scenario of "I had to use an adrenaline injection, put the oxygen mask and setup the BIPAP machine to save a patient's life…do you know how difficult the procedure is for removing sputum?" certainly seemed more exciting. Ninjja was sure that at the earliest available opportunity, the observations would convert to actions. Despite the good faith in which injections or BIPAP or something else would be administered, it would be precarious to restore the natural equilibrium in her father's fragile state.

Ninjja was glad that the doctor was still in discussion mode rather than in instruction mode. She mustered all her courage and made one last attempt at providing some context to the patient's condition. She started by reminding the doctor about his own counsel. "Doctor, do you remember when I came to you for a second opinion six months back? You mentioned that such patients are best handled in a home-care environment. You also mentioned that if the injection is administered, the patient gets habituated, and shunting between the hospital and home becomes a normal affair. I would like to avoid that situation." The doctor had a thinking frown and was stroking his chin.

Ninjja saw this as a sign that she was not completely off and continued, "Actually, he has been moving around in the house on his own. His blood pressure was normal, his body oxygen was not too bad (eighty-nine percent), and the pulse was fine, too. There was a lot of discomfort, but he was able to do his basic chores until two hours ago. To be honest, when he was released from the hospital after his bronchoscopy, he was in a much worse situation. He needed support for everything…and yet he stabilized at home."

The last line caught doctor's attention, and he became more malleable. He asked a few more questions and then said tentatively, "Well, if you have the oxygen machine at home and can arrange for BIPAP as needed, you can try to stabilize him at home." He prescribed a few medications and continued, "Call me tomorrow and tell me how he is doing." After a few other caveats and sundry instructions, the doctor asked the emergency staff to discharge the patient and signed off.

Ninjja said a genuine "Thank you" and proceeded to secure the release of her father.

Ninjja was met with sullen, grumpy faces. She had certainly hurt their egos (in addition to jeopardizing the revenue targets of the emergency room) and was in the line of fire now. The attending staff refused to acknowledge their guilt at disrupting the regulator of Ninjja's oxygen cylinder. However, her mother was not the type who would accept defeat. She managed to get one of the conscientious attendants to respond to her incessant pleas. He obliged by getting a sealing tape and plugging the leakage that was caused by disrespectful handling by the hospital staff. "It seems we did commit a major crime by getting our own equipment to the hospital. They would have annihilated this cylinder if they could…I am glad that it survived," Ninjja remarked to her mother.

"Yes, I can understand that they wouldn't want to use patient's equipment, the same way as your own food wouldn't be allowed in a restaurant; but such contemptuous handling is difficult to fathom," her mother responded in a distraught tone. While she was glad that Ninjja's father would not need to stay at the hospital, uncertainty was weighing on her mind.

"Father, how are you feeling now?" Ninjja tried to shift the focus back to the core issue.

He smiled feebly and said, "Better...I want to go home." Given the utter chaos and strain that he had been put through, such a response was a pleasant surprise. Possibly the strong nebulizer and high-pressure oxygen had more than compensated for the mayhem unleashed by the hospital staff.

"That's good news! I just need to pay the bill, and then we can leave," Ninjja responded in a reassuring tone.

However, the tunnel was much longer than what Ninjja had imagined. When the bill did not arrive even after a further wait of fifteen minutes, Ninjja started getting impatient. She wanted her father to be back in the comfortable environment of home. "Nurse, how long will it take? We have already been here for over two and half hours now," Ninjja called out to a nurse who was within audible range.

"Why don't you go and speak to the head of the emergency?" the nurse responded in a hurry and walked away. After several minutes of searching, when Ninjja finally located the head of emergency, she was met with an unwelcoming look. When she put forward her request for expediting her billing, the look turned into a glare that would have been enough to turn a slightly weak-spirited person into jelly. "There is a process, and it has to take the time it has to...I can't do much," he responded in a stern tone.

"Considering the state of the patient, it would be helpful if you could try to expedite the process." Ninjja tried to appear pleading and confident at the same time.

"First of all, you are making a big mistake by not admitting this patient to the hospital. It is a big risk, and I want you to sign an undertaking that you are taking him away at your own responsibility. You wasted our time." He paused to see if Ninjja was still standing on her two feet after this venomous sting.

Ninjja was certainly rattled but managed to conceal her true state. Was she indeed making a mistake? What if she was really risking her father's life? Ninjja was scared enough to question her decisions one more time. Her gut was telling her that in the current situation, the option of recuperating in a hospital bed was equivalent of leaving your car overnight at a local mechanic's workshop in India for minor vibrations. The chances that the whole suspension system would be opened up and all the car interiors soiled with grease without fixing the root cause were indeed high.

"Which papers do I need to sign, Doctor?" Ninjja gulped her anxieties and replied with a straight face. She had made her decision.

Two forms were shoved in front of her with utter disdain. By uniting her pen with the dotted line, Ninjja absolved the hospital of all their responsibilities and liabilities. The doctor snatched the papers and walked away with angry steps. Ninjja retraced her steps to her father, who was now trying to control his hunger pangs. A packet of biscuits in her all-encompassing purse came to the rescue.

Finally, the discharge bill arrived. Ninjja's jaw literally dropped. The bill ran into few pages and totaled to Rs. 10,000 (US$200), twenty times the regular consultation charges of Rs. 500 (US$10). Ninjja was mentally prepared for a multiple of four to five, given that they had consulted with the doctor in an emergency room, and there was an X-ray and a blood sample taken. As Ninjja stared at the bill with her eyes popping out, the image of the young lady doctor with her unstoppable list of tests flashed through her mind. "Oh, my God! Looks like all the blood tests on planet Earth were ordered!" In addition to the tests, there were multiple charges for consultations with all the doctors that had made an appearance. Exorbitant charges for the oxygen, nebulization, and sundry disposable items (like the oxygen mask) were the topping on this broth that had cooked over the past three hours. It was too thick for Ninjja's liking, but she had no energy left to question the ingredients anymore and gulped it down without any further protests. "Can I get the reports, please?" was the only one-liner that found its way out.

The reply was, "You can collect them tomorrow afternoon."

This time around, Ninjja got introduced to one more variety of doctor in the form of the emergency-room head, and she couldn't help giving him a name! He was "Docboon," who thought that he was the biggest gift to the mankind. He juggled many patients and was extremely loyal to "SOULMAC."

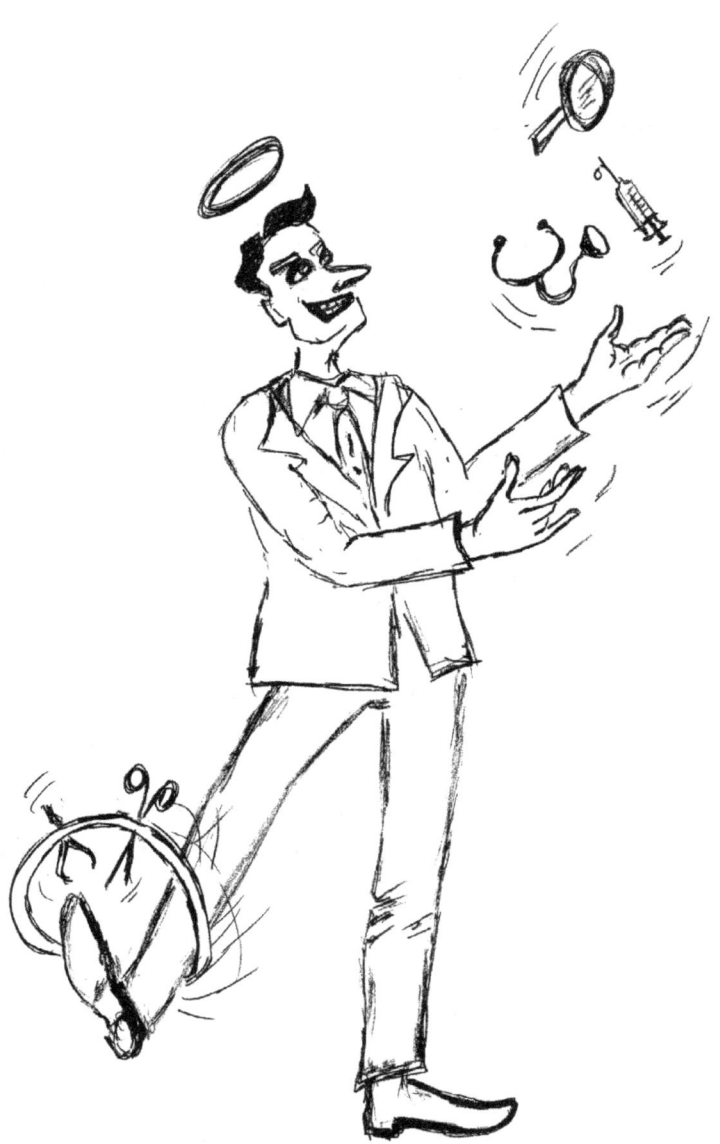

Docboon: Thinks he is the biggest gift to mankind. Juggles many patients and is extremely loyal to SOULMAC

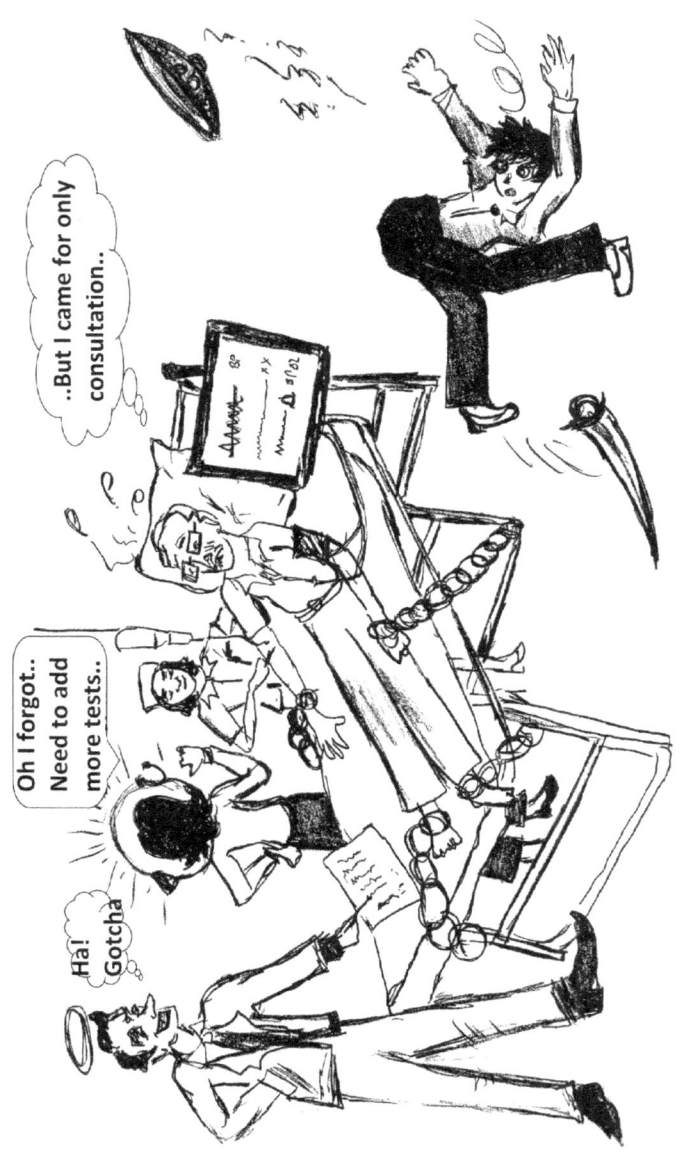

Emergency room: Terror Unleashed!

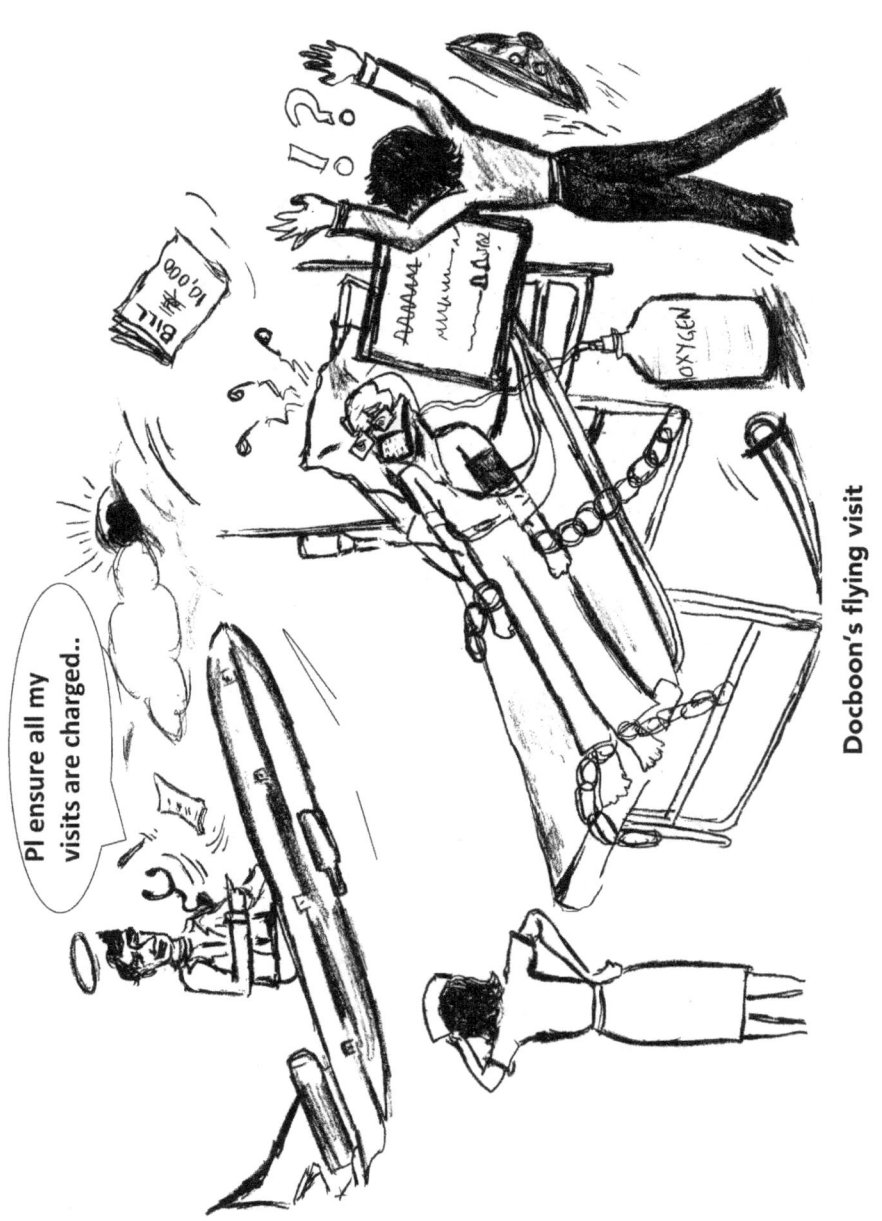

Docboon's flying visit

While she was walking in, perhaps she had forgotten that every-thing was being governed by "SOULMAC

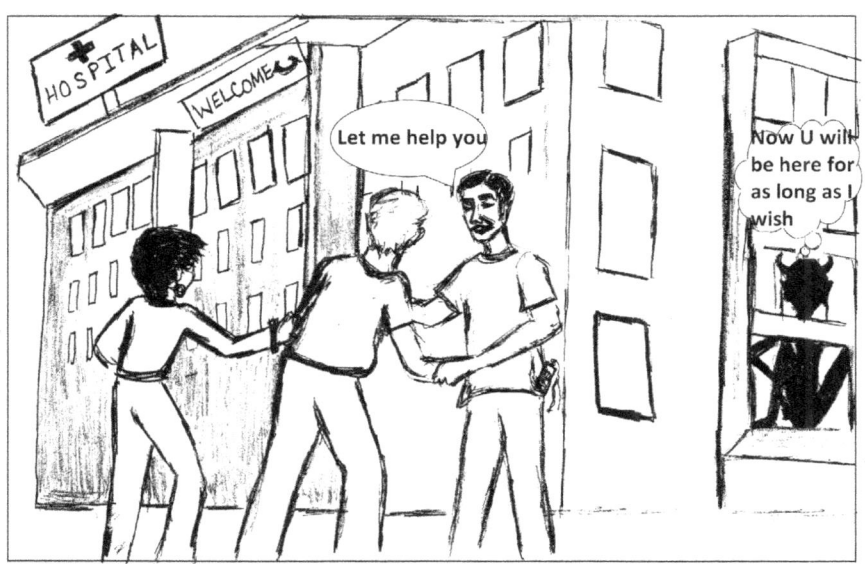

Ninjja at the hospital gate

• • •

Once they were home, the simple home food, a few hours of sleep, and new medication had already started having some positive im-pact. The following day, Ninjja's father reported that he was feeling much better. Ninjja wondered if the dreadful experience of the pre-vious day had rejuvenated his determination to recover faster and avoid another trip to the hospital at any cost.

• • •

Ninjja decided to step out of the office during her lunch break to collect the reports and run them by the doctor.

She offered the thick envelope of reports for his review. The doctor could not conceal his surprise, and his instant reaction was "Oh, they got so many tests done..." He flipped through the pages in a few seconds and stopped on a couple of sheets to really read something. "There is no need to worry. There is an infection, but the antibiotics should be able to take care of it."

It was clear to Ninjja that the bulk of the tests were redundant from the patient's perspective but clearly profitable for the hospital. Ninjja thanked the doctor and politely slipped in some feedback about the ordeal and financial damage at the emergency room the previous day. Ninjja could sense that the doctor was embarrassed and wanted to avoid the topic. At least the system was not expected to run this way. She was glad that someone felt a tad embarrassed that they had let the patient down.

Once there was a sense that things were under control, she could look back over the events of the past twenty-four hours with amusement. Ninjja was amazed at both the flexibility and the fragility of the human mind. The same events that generated anger, anxiety, and frustration were, with a change in time and space, now creating amusement. Ninjja was keen to share the narrative with someone and dialed Arv's number, hoping that he would still be on his extended lunch break.

"Oh, hello...where have you been?" he answered.

"Well, acting in a hospital drama...but fortunately, I could write my own dialogue and force some changes to the script," Ninjja replied, smiling.

"Tell me more," Arv responded with interest, propelling her to continue.

Before she put the phone down, Ninjja thanked Arv and said, "I want you to know that your philosophy of 'natural equilibrium' was ringing in my head constantly. That really helped me with taking a tough stand. I just hope that I am right!"

After a week, kudos from the doctor on seeing marked improvement in her father's mental and physical health provided the affirmation that Ninjja was looking for.

That night, Ninjja had a good reason to pull out her yellow diary again.

―⁂―

My Survival Mantra

1. Don't assume that your regular physician will always know what is right for you.
2. When in doubt, seek a second opinion.
3. Always have health insurance, and carefully select the plan.
4. Don't rush to a specialist based on your perceived issue.
5. Overseas insurance is not a blank check.
6. A balanced lifestyle holds the secret of many a cure.
7. In emergency situations (e.g., an accident), don't run to the closest hospital.
8. If someone dear to you is admitted to the hospital, don't assume that the nurses and attendants are always right.

9. Several diseases may have stress as the underlying cause.
10. Watch out for medicine addiction!
11. Emotional support is a substitute for some medicines.
12. Don't take medicines in blind faith.
13. There is no utopian health-care system.
14. Childhood diet and lifestyle define a large portion of adult health.
15. Explore alternative therapies before going under the knife if you are not in a time-critical situation.
16. Think before you start making all your health issues public.
17. **Proactively share and challenge the context, especially for older patients.** Based on pure looks and vitals, it is more likely that the older patients will look much paler, weaker, and in worse shape than their younger counterparts. While some discerning doctors would be able to make the right call (adjusting for the age factor) about admission to the hospital, relying on luck alone can't be the answer! It is well proven that hospitals (and especially ICUs) are responsible for several infections that can further complicate an older patient's recovery. Any uncalled-for hospital admission would be exposing the older patient to further risks. It is important to have a good understanding of historical instances and the patient's response/recovery model. More importantly, openly sharing it with the attending doctors is even more critical.

Remember, there is no need to jump into the water if you don't know how to swim... and if you need to, make sure that you are at the shallow end of the pool.

⁓

. . .

A cool breeze in the morning signaled that there might be some relief from the blistering heat during the day. Ninjja was having a quick breakfast when her father found a moment to talk to her. "Can you take your mother to the hospital?" he hesitatingly said, ignoring the glaring eyes of her mother. The glare meant that her mother did not want him to add more burdens to Ninjja's already crowded portfolio. "Why, what's wrong?" Ninjja asked hurriedly.

"There is a huge blister on your mother's back, and it is growing more painful by the day," he responded.

Ninjja managed to convince her reluctant father that it was fine to go along with the driver for this. "Don't you worry...this is not something for which they will put her into an emergency room," Ninjja told him jokingly.

As she stepped out, she couldn't help wondering how the recent episodes of hospital visits had made her father paranoid to the point that he was scared to visit a hospital alone.

As it turned out, the issue wasn't that simple after all. It did require a minor procedure, and the attending doctor recommended couple of days of hospital stay! The suggestion was nothing short of a huge tide that inundated the delicately balanced ship of Ninjja's household. Till this point it had never occurred to Ninjja how hard things could get for an older couple. If one of the two was in need of constant care, there was no space for any medical emergency for the other person. The good news was that in the Indian context, personal relationships did offer some latitude.

The specialist who was attending to Ninjja's father came to the rescue. In response to his request, the doctor altered the procedure he was planning for her mother. It meant a longer time for healing and multiple visits to the hospital for follow-ups, but it saved her from staying at the hospital.

Ninjja hated to see her father's helplessness. She could see that he really wanted to accompany her mother for every hospital visit, but his propensity to catch infections prohibited him from doing so.

"I feel so useless...I can do nothing for your mother," he finally said in a dejected tone. "Actually, no one even asks for my point of view."

This was a poignant moment for Ninjja. Her father's physical limitations hadn't constrained his desire to care for his loved ones. So far, it had never occurred to Ninjja that the constant attention and care that her father was receiving, combined with his inability to give back, also acted as a heavy burden on his weak shoulders. Someone who was used to being a shield for the whole family was now reduced to being the delicate entity that had to be protected! *How unnerving and frustrating this must be*, Ninjja thought, and she gulped to find her vocal chords, as something needed to be said. "You are thinking about her, and you want to be there with her...this thought itself is enough. You don't need to feel bad. I know that your thoughts are already offering her enough strength." Ninjja made a vain attempt to comfort him.

Learned and sensitive man that he was, he decided to humor Ninjja and settled back in his study chair on the pretext of writing something.

That night, Ninjja went to bed with the guilt of someone who had inadvertently incarcerated someone. She couldn't keep herself away from her yellow diary and scribbled, "In your zest for caring for an incapacitated loved one, don't undermine their sense of pride and freedom to decide. The love and care is worthwhile only to the extent that it doesn't smother them."

·   ·   ·

SEPTEMBER 2011

It was Ninjja's father's seventy-sixth birthday. He had been on an upward trajectory for the past few months and was in great spirits for the celebration. He was happy that the jinx of seventy-five that ran in his family had been broken. Ninjja learned later that the paranoia that her father had experienced during periods of bad health was partly due to the fact that everyone in his family had died at the age of seventy-five. "The period of danger is finally over," he muttered with a mystical glint in his eyes.

They had an amalgamation of the East and the West in their celebrations—a cake combined with Hindu customs. Ninjja's father couldn't wait to try on the pair of suspenders that Ninjja brought for him as a birthday gift. He was so sporting that he wore them around his portly form without any hesitation and took full interest in posing for the photo ops that Ninjja was conducting.

Technology made it possible to share the pictures instantly with her sister, and the stimulating comments from the other end added the final garnish to an already appealing entrée.

"Father, in few weeks you will gain more strength, and the weather will also get better. We will go to Akshardham...the temple that you always wanted to visit." Ninjja didn't need to wait for a verbal response. The shine in his eyes told her that this was the best birthday present that he could have asked for.

Suddenly, the computer buzzed, and there was the little angel on the other end wishing her grandpa a very happy birthday. The lisp in the booming voice of Ninjja's little niece felt like music. "Chylender (Cylinder) Baba...happy birthday," she cooed with a bright smile. "I want to come to India..." Her chatter continued, with only a third of it decipherable. However, the communication between the grandparents and the grandchild wasn't dependent on the words. Ninjja was amused to see how happy both sides looked. Indeed, this was the perfect ending to a great celebration.

• • •

NOVEMBER 2011

A wedding was announced in the family. Suddenly, the upcoming great Indian wedding had become the fulcrum around which all the dinner-table discussions revolved. Unknowingly, the annoying topics of medication, issues with attendants, and visits to the doctors had found their way under the carpet and had made space for more pleasant topics. A few days later, Ninjja's cousin came in to personally extend the invitation. The warmth and sincerity with which he urged them to come over twisted her tongue, and she blurted out, "Yes, I will definitely be there" instead of her usual "I will try my best to take some time off then."

Her dad's excitement was rising with every passing day. After all, his favorite grandchild was getting married. However, Ninjja wasn't prepared when her father announced, "We will all go together for the wedding." Ninjja and her mother both looked at him, eyes widened with shock and surprise. They just stopped short of saying, "Are you out of your mind?"

"Father, we are talking of a ninety-minute flight and at least six hours of total journey here...where will you find the energy to tolerate this ordeal?" Ninjja finally said.

"Don't you worry. I am perfectly fine now. I can go. I have also talked to the doctor, and he said it's OK for me to travel," he said with an almost childlike eagerness. Ninjja was spellbound with his enthusiasm.

"OK, let's think about it some more...the event is still more than a month away." Ninjja used the standard delaying tactic that she had seen in practice at many companies and government departments when they wanted to be polite in saying no.

Ninjja's father was also a master player of this game that she had just started. He didn't take her head-on but instead started offering snippets of his new feats, like climbing stairs and longer walks, as certificates of his perfect health. Ninjja couldn't help being impressed. His persistence and the daily conversations made her realize that, apart from the happiness of an important event, this was an occasion for him to meet all the people he cared about in the extended family. She couldn't bear to play him anymore and decided to put things straight after a fortnight.

"Father, I know that you would love to go there, and everyone in the family will be very happy to see you...but you must realize that this is very risky. We can't afford to expend all the recovery you have had in past few months in a jiffy. To be honest, I don't even know if airlines allow transportation of oxygen machines. You are in a comfort zone here where everything, including your diet, is specially designed for you…how will we replicate it in a different city for just few days? What if there is a medical emergency? The new doctors will have no idea of your case history…I hope you understand."

Her father was unmoved. "I am absolutely doing fine. I can stay without this oxygen machine for ten hours at a stretch if I want to," he replied with a confidence that Ninjja had forgotten about.

It looked like this was a thing he absolutely had to do if he were to ever live happily. Ninjja couldn't muster up the courage to say that she wouldn't even try.

She picked up the phone to talk to the airlines with the feeling that someone around her was determined to commit hara-kiri, and she had no control over it. Ninjja started going through the motions of dialing various numbers to get through to someone who could answer her queries, but she seemed to be caught in an infinite loop. The elapsed time started bringing back her concerns to the fore, and suddenly all the waiting on the phone started appearing meaningless. An airplane clearly qualified to be in the category of enclosed public spaces where infections had ample opportunities to spread. Given the 100 percent track record of her father falling sick after previous visits to the malls, Ninjja almost got a panic attack.

*How naïve of me! Why did I even try to call the airlines? What if the person on the next seat is sneezing or has the flu…or…*Ninjja's mind was racing fast, and she concluded that this was the worst possible idea for humoring her father.

"I can't let you jump into a well while I am watching. I will not be able to forgive myself," Ninjja announced to her father with a sinking feeling. "I feel that I am reasoning with a small child who is fixated on having the neighbor's toy. Please try to understand…" Ninjja tried her best to explain the logic and the risks one more time. She painfully watched her father's cheerful face lose its hue with each passing sentence.

He finally spoke slowly, "OK. So be it. Why don't you at least take your mother with you?"

Ninjja saw this as a signal that his positive spirit was still breathing and responded with all excitement, "I am sure we can work on this. I could stay with you, and she can go…" The feeling that he was chaining Ninjja's mother to home due to his own disability was probably a bigger driver for his immovable urge than his own desire to socialize.

The countdown to D-day had begun, when something unexpected happened. One of Ninjja's close uncles suddenly passed away. He had just returned from an exciting, multidestination vacation when a massive heart attack claimed its superiority over his vivacity.

Ninjja's mother wanted to run to her sister in a jiffy and offer her whatever consolation was possible in that situation.

After several deliberations and carefully masking the true situation from her father, Ninjja's mother decided to take off with a heavy heart. This was her first flight alone…ever.

Ninjja was confident that she would be able to handle the situation at home with the able support of her father's attendant. He was a skilled and intelligent worker, whenever he wasn't absent on the pretext of illness. It was difficult to fathom that every month, some illness bestowed itself upon him or one of his family members; but Ninjja's family was willing to overlook his absenteeism, considering his other good qualities. Ninjja was hopeful that he would be available as he was just back from a week long disappearance.

Ninjja wasn't sure if her father had fallen for the explanation that her uncle was in the hospital or whether he was just playing along. Whatever the truth was, he looked deeply concerned. He kept enquiring about her uncle's health every few hours and then finally raised a red flag. "I think something is wrong! Why is no one answering my phone?"

Ninjja was caught off guard.

She hadn't thought of the possibility that her father would start his own investigation so soon. "Well, they must be all worked up... how do you expect people waiting on a serious patient at the hospital to answer phones?" She tried a weak argument.

Her first day alone with her father started off well, with all the support staff reporting on time. Her father thoroughly savored every bite of the stuffed paratha (a form of Indian bread) she made and said it was a welcome change from the bland meals that he was being served day after day. Culinary experimentation was not something that Ninjja's mother enjoyed; she was happy delivering the standard, time-tested products to the submissive patient. They exchanged a few jokes on this topic and were happy to discover that his life was not all that constrained after all. The avenue of enjoying food was still open to her father, provided someone in charge showed some latitude.

However hard Ninjja tried to work from home that day, she couldn't avoid stepping out for few hours for a critical meeting. However, she wasn't worried. The skilled attendant was on duty and had given her his full assurance that he would be watching her dad like a hawk.

Three hours later, Ninjja was back. She rang the bell. When the door wasn't opened for five minutes, she reached for the doorbell for a second time.

A worried Ninjja had extended her hand for a third time when she heard some footsteps approaching the door from inside the house. After a lot of clunking and swooshing, the door finally opened, and there was her father, looking visibly tired. He was clearly out of practice with opening the main door with its multiple locking mechanisms.

"Father, why did you answer the door? Where is our man?" Ninjja was surprised.

"He doesn't seem normal. He is not responding to me properly and has been falling asleep intermittently," Ninjja's father responded in a suspicious tone. He looked more intrigued than really concerned. "OK. Watch me. I will show you." He moved with a childlike curiosity to show off his new discovery. He proceeded to the room where the attendant was blissfully snoozing in a chair, completely unaware of the approaching footsteps. Ninjja's father mustered his full strength to call out his name and said, "Are you all right? Wake up." Getting no response, he nudged him gently with his stick and softly whispered to Ninjja, "See, now he will wake up."

Sure enough, the attendant stirred a bit, opened his eyes, and blabbered, "Sorry...I dozed off...don't know what has gone wrong today..."

It took Ninjja's stern voice to shake him up from his slumber and spring him back on his feet. "Have you come here after doing night duty at the hospital? I will need to call your supervisor!" Ninjja was fuming now.

"No, no, madam, don't do that," the attendant started pleading. Ninjja could now clearly see that his eyes were red, and his tongue was slurring. "This doesn't look like a case of an overworked man." Ninjja exchanged a meaningful glance with her father. She continued the conversation to test the slurring and the general motor control.

After watching his unsteady steps she instinctively remarked, "I think he is drunk! What do you say, Father?"

"I have the same feeling, but I can't imagine how," he responded in a brooding tone.

"You need to ask him directly and confront him." In socially accepted norms, confronting a drunk man fell more in the domain of a man than a woman.

While the confrontation didn't elicit any incriminating evidence, unknowingly, several new facts unfolded themselves. The fact that the attendant was in possession of the keys to her father's two-wheeler along with a sizeable amount of money pointed her ire in the direction of her father now. "What were you thinking?

What was the need to dole out all these goodies to him?" she snapped.

"I wanted him to get some fruit…thought it would be much faster if he had a vehicle!" her guileless father responded sheepishly.

"So where is the fruit?" She looked around, trying to control the volcano that was brewing inside her.

"He said the fruit was of pathetic quality, so he didn't bring any," her father replied. "I suppose that excuse was fishy."

"And I am sure that he didn't return the money that was never spent? We at least now know the window of opportunity he has had for his little escapade. Has he been this way ever since he got back?"

Her father paused to think. "Well, no…he was fine when he got back. For the past hour or so, he has been behaving oddly."

"Hmm…we need to get the truth from him!" Ninjja wasn't prepared to stop until there was a confession. "I think we need to get someone who is more experienced in this matter," she continued and walked across the hallway to see if their neighbor was home. Fortunately, he was back and gladly obliged.

Several Machiavellian moves later, the neighbor declared success! He had managed to extract all the details of this little escapade, including the empty bottle of cheap country liquor that was carefully hidden in a shelf in the storeroom. The attendant also begged for forgiveness, claiming that this was the first time that he had indulged himself while on duty. Clearly, the absence of the lady with the iron hand had given him the false sense of comfort that he was a free bird!

Ninjja tried her best at tact to extract the keys to the vehicle from his possession. A few minutes later, with the keys carefully tucked away in the drawer, she packed off the attendant for good. As she slumped back into the sofa, all the missing links started falling into place. The mystery of long absenteeism had a plausible explanation now. It was the impact of excesses with cheap country liquor that had incapacitated this attendant for long periods of time. Ninjja was appalled as well as saddened—appalled at the complete lapse of background checks by the hospital's agency and saddened at the prospect of a skilled, intelligent, poor man creating and riding his own path of destruction. She called the person in charge of the agency in a fit of angst.

"How can you send people with a drinking problem to take care of patients that need home care? Do you do any background checks? We had a situation where the patient was looking after the attendant! What if my father had needed some emergency support?" Her voice trailed off in despair. Once her need for venting was fulfilled, she disconnected the phone.

Two days later, Ninjja's mother was back home. In the meanwhile, through a gradual unfolding of facts, her father had come to know of her uncle's demise. Despite his challenges with depression and ill health, he accepted the news gracefully as the ultimate truth that everyone should be ready to face. Ninjja was amazed at his poise and ability to appreciate the surreal while being totally oblivious to even simple connivances of daily life.

There was no news from the attendant or his agency. As the payment was required to be made in advance, the responsibility of extracting the right services from the agency naturally fell upon the family of the needy patient. Ninjja was surprised that word of mouth and continuity of services had no place in the current thinking of the service providers.

. . .

Four days later, an unexpected visitor turned up: the attendant.

His wife was standing few steps behind him with her head bowed down. She looked to be a simple, semiurban lady who was embarrassed at her husband's behavior. The attendant started apologizing profusely and accepted that he was grappling with a drinking problem.

His wife was almost in tears at her inability to correct the situation. Her story of constant struggle with managing finances and the responsibility of her six-month-old baby was indeed moving. With great difficulty, Ninjja managed to maintain a tough posture and expressed her inability to engage a drunkard to take care of her ill father. However, at the same time, she was moved to see the agony of this family that had the capacity of leading a good life. She couldn't avoid getting into counseling mode.

"You are multiskilled and are a fast learner—I hope you know that! If you focus on any field where you want to stick around, you will be in great demand. You can provide a good life to your family…why would you not want to do that? I am sure your well-to-do father didn't imagine your life would pan out like this." Ninjja tried to remind him of the historical facts to reinforce the message. His body language indicated that her input was being absorbed.

"Madam, what should I do? I have been trying very hard, but I end up succumbing to the bottle if I see one," he responded genuinely. Ninjja knew that professional rehab services would be beyond the means of this poor man, so she tried to look for easier solutions by talking more.

"When do you see a bottle that you can't resist?"

"Whenever I am with my friends," he responded innocently.

"Are you saying that you don't drink alone?" Ninjja didn't want to believe him.

"The episode starts with drinking with friends...then sometimes I continue alone on subsequent days," he confessed with his head down.

Ninjja could find this more believable based on the incident that she had witnessed four days ago.

"Would you meet me if you knew that I would serve you poison-laced drink?" Ninjja continued with a dramatic tone for a better impact. The attendant looked perplexed. "You have to imagine that all these friends of yours are keen to poison you. The only way that you can escape this disastrous addiction of yours is if you stop meeting these friends," Ninjja opined with a conviction of a judge. Her charged discourse seemed to have struck a chord with the attendant. Her parents chipped in with their anecdotes and words of wisdom. His wife was looking at Ninjja and her parents with hopeful eyes. There was tentativeness in Ninjja's eyes when she returned her glance. She did not want to give a false sense of hope to the poor woman.

"I promise you—I won't meet these friends at all. I am ashamed of myself." The attendant spoke slowly.

"Well, this has to come from within you; the rest of your family can just provide you support. If you really want to do this, in addition to avoiding these friends like plague, please make sure that you don't have any cash on you. We wish you good luck for your fight." Ninjja hoped that they would leave now.

"Uncle, I want my job back. Please allow me to come back here. I assure you, I won't give you a chance to be upset ever again." The attendant now appealed to her father's kindness.

"First, you have to prove that you are through with your addiction. We can't take any more risks," Ninjja came in firmly. However, that was not an answer that was going to go down that easily. The attendant kept elaborating on his desperate situation, and his wife supported him fully with intermittent showers of tears.

It did look like the agency had taken some action on her complaint. They had simply fired the attendant, without offering him any support to fight his drinking problem. Though it did not absolve the agency of the grievous risks that they were exposing the patients to, at least it did point to some sort of an internal feedback mechanism.

Ninjja was getting incredibly late for work, but the story of inordinate misery combined with a bucketful of tears had already started melting her soft-hearted father. "Please give me a second chance!" the attendant pleaded.

"We have already suffered through several periods of your unannounced absence…you had given us enough of false stories. You have already received many more chances." Ninjja was determined not to budge.

"It seems that he has acknowledged the root cause of his problem. Now he is at least promising to work on it," Ninjja's father said to Ninjja in their native tongue. He was softened by the overflowing emotions as well as his own fondness for the attendant, who had endeared himself more as a friend than just a service provider. The attendant's skills and good nature weren't lost on Ninjja, but given the potential of high risks, she was inclined to take a very tough stand. Ninjja's mother agreed with her.

Finally, a few internal conferences and some more tears later, the family gave in.

"Look, this is absolutely your last chance! We will be watching you very closely. You need to get my mother's permission every time you need to step out, and you need to show her all the medication before administering it. Is that absolutely clear? Any slipup, and there will be no further discussion. If this is fine with you, I will speak to the agency and ask them to send you back," Ninjja said firmly.

She secretly hoped that this last chance was something that would do the magic trick to turn this person around. She was pained to see that someone with such high potential could go to waste without another chance. Fortunately, her father was in a state where he needed a companion to talk to constantly rather than really a caregiver. Ninjja hoped that her father's tremendous knowledge, which shined through all the dialogues (or monologues, at times), would have an effect on the attendant. Though it was a tricky decision, there was a sense of satisfaction and hope.

That night Ninjja went to bed feeling positive despite the fairly unnerving episode that had unfolded over the last few days. Her father was happy, as was evident from the dinner-table stories that he shared with her. Her mother's accounts gave testimony to the commitment and alertness of the attendant. Ninjja reached out for her yellow diary to jot down another challenge that was staring at the health-care system, especially in the developing countries.

—ᴍ—

A receiver's perspective on health-care challenges

1. Death of the quintessential family doctor
2. Moral corruption spreading its wings in the medical profession
3. Affordability of health-care
4. Quality of attendants and nurses
5. Availability and credibility of information on alternative cures
6. Indiscreet use and abuse of health-care reimbursements and insurance
7. **Primitive home-care services**

   Increasing average life span, reducing family size, and increasing numbers of women joining the workforce in developing countries mean that there will be more older people who need health-care workers to support them at home. Unfortunately, it looks like the whole system is caught napping. Four pieces of the jigsaw puzzle don't lend themselves to easy maneuvering:

- <u>Mind-sets</u>: The upcoming generations of septuagenarians don't realize that they won't have an extended family in the house to look after them and hence are ill pre-pared emotionally as well as financially for external help.

- <u>Unskilled workforce</u>: Given the general absence of lower-middle-class educated workers, almost anyone who has been to a primary school is considered fit enough to serve as a home health-care worker and is expected to learn at the expense of unsus-pecting patients. Unfortunately, little is done to upgrade their skill sets. Any sane mind would be shocked to learn that a health-care attendant who can't read English (which is the language for writing prescrip-tions) can survive the system. Needless to say, a background check falls much lower in the pecking order! To top it all, even if a skilled person is found, he or she might be debilitated due to social challenges (e.g., drinking problems, abusive household); and if the employment agency doesn't provide a support mechanism to such individuals, the patient is likely to bear the brunt of all lapses. Such an appalling lack of skills can surely inspire fear in a few early adopters and jeopardize the long-term development of a much-needed service.

- <u>Pricing challenges</u>: Despite a monthly billing rate for customers that typically exceeds the pension of any middle-class retiree, the service providers don't want to increase the salary that they offer their employees, which jeopardizes any chances of finding the right talent; and they are not ready to invest in training and upgrading their skill levels. The challenge being quoted is economics. High levels of attrition, management costs, and variable utilization levels act as a drag on their profits. From a patient's affordability perspective, clearly there doesn't seem any room for prices to go further north unless there is some sort of financial support coming through either insurance or the government. Even if some support were to come through, how could such a steep price point for such a shoddy service be justified?

- <u>Accountability and processes for quality control</u>: The problem of shoddy service can't be entirely blamed on the poor skill level of staff. Given the sheer dearth of branded service providers, the demand continues to overshadow the need for proving accountability. With minimal processes for quality control, agencies can be in business as long as they have some basic business ethics, such as not disappearing overnight after the advance has been collected! The presence of several unscrupulous operators makes providers of "just the warm bodies that do show up" shine in comparison. Being accountable for not having a person with a drinking addiction for health-care support would not even be up for debate elsewhere in the developed world!

—︎m—

While she was busy intellectualizing this challenge, some elderly person who wasn't fortunate enough to have his or her family maintain closer control was probably suffering at the hands of an ill-equipped health-care worker somewhere in this country!

"At a minimum, people should be aware of the gaping holes before they find themselves stuck in them," she signed off in her diary, hoping that she could start an awareness campaign at the least.

. . .

One month later, the circle of life continued to spin. It was now time for the wedding! The celebrations were on, albeit in a subdued manner.

Ninjja also joined the wedding, without her parents. She was missing her father, especially considering his childlike yearning to meet everyone. "Oh, I wish I could do something," she told one of her cousins. Suddenly a brain wave struck her.

"Why can't I use technology?" she exclaimed and got up in excitement. "I just hope that Mother is able to use all the technology training I have been forcibly giving her over the years," she muttered as she dialed her number.

Ninjja's mother proved her meticulousness once again. She followed the step-by-step instructions that she had jotted down in her notebook and was on Skype in less than ten minutes. Ninjja's iPhone had a good 3G signal all through the wedding venue, and in no time, her father was watching the wedding live as well as talking to his extended family. He was elated. The tinkle in his voice, the shine in his eyes, and the smile on his face were absolutely priceless. The creators of technology may not have thought about the "gift of smile" that they unknowingly created for humankind. She silently thanked these "nuovo gods" and watched the proceedings with contentment.

.   .   .

Three weeks later, Ninjja's sister and little niece were keeping her father fully entertained, while the illustrious attendant had fallen prey to his addiction yet again.

After another of his unannounced, weeklong disappearances, Ninjja's father stayed true to their earlier conversations and dismissed him without another word. Ninjja's hopes of being a social reformer were quashed to the ground! The fact that the family had grown attached to this man, and they couldn't do anything to stop the rollercoaster ride of his self-destruction, caused them more pain.

Ninjja's father surprised her once again by his poise and offered her one more important philosophical sound bite: "If a body part can't be cured, it needs to be cut off to save a life...one needs to focus on the life that is being saved rather than the loss of the body part. If he were to continue being a health-care attendant without mending his ways, he would be putting many lives at risk...so let it go," he continued in the same breath.

• • •

JANUARY 2012

The winter had reached its peak, with bone-chilling winds and minimum temperatures nearing the freezing mark. Fortunately, the new technology of the hot-and-cold air conditioner was delivering on its promise. Ninjja was glad to see that her father was doing well, unlike the previous winter, when his condition had significantly deteriorated despite a heavy dosage of steroids.

It was time to bid adieu to Ninjja's sister. The emotions were difficult to contain. Ninjja could see them streaming out of her father's eyes when her sister hugged him tightly. "Be careful. Take good care of yourself and your family." He made a parting remark with great difficulty.

Ninjja tried to lighten up the mood by saying, "Don't you know that things are the other way around here? The little one takes care of your daughter..." She pointed a finger at her sister and continued, "Don't you worry; she will be back soon to get all the pampering from you." Neither of them reacted, possibly due to the invisible wall of uncertainty that lay between them.

The affection between father and daughter did not need any words. Neither spoke, but the way they were holding hands said it all. The clock was ticking, and both were hoping that the other one would let go first. The image of her sister's soft, small palms clutching onto her father's weatherworn, thin, wrinkled hands was imprinted in Ninjja's memory. The pain of separation and doubts about the next meeting were visible in her father's large, beautiful, sea-blue eyes.

"Ajoba [Granddad], Aai [Mother]—don't be sad. I get sad, too. We need to go in aeloplane[airplane]. My baba [dad] is waiting," spoke her niece with a long, innocent face. Her display of newly acquired language skills was impressive, and more importantly, it created a welcome distraction.

The weather was too severe for Ninjja's father to come to the airport, so he had to be content with an hour less with the daughter he liked to pamper the most.

Ninjja was reminded of the days when her father used to run with the train even beyond the main platform while seeing her off during her college days. He did not want to miss even a split-second glimpse of his daughter till it was humanly impossible. Ninjja couldn't believe that she was staring at the same person.

During their drive to the airport, Ninjja's niece lifted up their spirits with her incessant chatter and made the good-byes more perfunctory than emotional.

•   •   •

Three weeks later, Ninjja noticed that her father was not looking too well. Upon inquiry, she learned that he was suffering from severe back pain. "Since when?" she asked.

"It has been seven or eight days," her mother responded.

"I also spoke to the doctor, and he has increased the steroids to forty milligrams," added her father.

"What? You have suddenly gone from fifteen to forty? And for back pain? Your breathing seems fine...I don't see the logic of increasing steroids meant for COPD for a problem with the back!" Ninjja reacted peevishly.

"I felt the same…that's why I have increased to only thirty," Ninjja's mother jumped in.

"But why didn't you at least tell me? Maybe the doctor did not understand him properly on the phone. Maybe he thought that the breathing had become worse due to the severe winter."

There was complete silence. She realized that her parents hadn't wanted to bother her, taking cognizance of the grueling schedule that she had been keeping. Ninjja forced her father to call the doctor again to reconfirm the course of medication. After watching her father meander around the problem for few minutes, Ninjja grabbed the phone from him in frustration. She articulated the situation to the best of her abilities and waited for an answer.

"Oh! I thought that he was suffering from breathing trouble, which is very common in this month for such patients," came the reply, proving Ninjja's fears. "But I don't think you should reduce the dosage now. For the back pain, he can take…" the doctor advised, while Ninjja tried hard to jot down the unpronounceable spellings.

Ninjja gave an annoyed glance to her parents. "How could you be so naïve? You have taken a much heavier dosage for the past week when this was not needed! Now the doctor has asked us to continue steroids at the same level…it seems odd, but I don't know any better." Ninjja seemed to be at the end of her patience. Her father now bore a scared expression, compelling her to soften her stand and add a few comforting words. "Don't worry. In a week or two, your dosage will be back to normal. In the meanwhile, also try the home remedies, like a hot oil wrap. You will be fine soon." She tried to hide her exasperation and smiled.

Days passed by, but the back pain showed no signs of improvement. Her father started looking more worried and harried and started getting alarmed at the slightest provocation. Her father's physiotherapist started worrying if there was a fracture. However, it wasn't easy to validate his suspicion.

Ninjja didn't think he would be able to withstand the three-hour ordeal of visiting an orthopedic and getting an X-ray or CT scan done. As Ninjja had painfully learned the last time around, it was impossible to get any doctor to pay a home visit. Finally, Ninjja decided to take a favor from a very experienced orthophysiotherapist whom she knew. He obliged.

· · ·

The family was pleased to know that there was absolutely no possibility of a fracture. The physiotherapist suggested a treatment that needed specific equipment. However, he was wise enough to judge the reality of the situation and didn't think it was advisable for Ninjja's father to travel to a clinic to undergo therapy.

"I will try to send someone from my team tomorrow to start the basic exercises…and in the meanwhile, I will scour around for a portable machine that we need." The last sentence offered a lot of comfort, but before they could thank him, Ninjja's father jumped in with a desperate plea: "Doctor, please, I want you to come tomorrow. I want no one else." His eagerness and desperation seemed a bit embarrassing. However, the senior physiotherapist took it very well and proceeded to comfort him. Ninjja was impressed to see his patience and skill of counseling that was rare to find even in psychiatrists. Later, he spoke to Ninjja in private. "He does look a bit paranoid. And also depressed. I think you should consult a psychiatrist."

"Yeah, I had the same feeling. I was thinking of taking him, once he gets some relief from the back pain," Ninjja concurred.

True to his word, the physiotherapist managed to arrange a portable machine, as well as appointed an experienced member of his team for treatment. Also, he kept his promise of visiting her father every alternate day. His prowess of speech possibly helped more than the core skill of physiotherapy at this juncture. In four or five days, the back pain had lessened considerably, confirming that the treatment being given was on the right track. However, the paranoia and confusion that her father was experiencing seemed to have increased considerably.

It was painful for Ninjja to watch her father go into panic mode with the most normal of routine things, like someone paying a visit without prior notice, the attendant getting delayed by a few minutes, kids screaming at the playground, or the maid not following instructions. Ninjja was convinced that medical intervention was needed, but given the criticality of his respiratory disease, it was not desirable to give any psychiatric medicines without the approval of the pulmonary specialist.

•   •   •

With great difficulty, Ninjja managed to get the stars aligned for the two doctors at the hospital to adjust their mutually exclusive visiting hours to accommodate her dad. Finally, they were sitting face-to-face with the pulmonary specialist, in whom her father had an almost religious faith despite the initial fiasco of the bronchoscopy. After examining him, the specialist pronounced that this was a steroid-induced paranoia/psychosis.

"He has been on a high dosage for too long," the doctor pronounced. Ninjja was perplexed, as the dosage was dramatically increased only as per the doctor's advice.

"Our first priority is to save life, that is, breathing; and only after that do we need to worry about dealing with these aftereffects," the doctor replied calmly as Ninjja looked on, puzzled.

However, in this latest context, the same old logic did not seem very convincing. The dosage was increased preemptively without any symptoms of breathing trouble. Even though there had been a misunderstanding in the telephone communication, there had been a window for course correction when Ninjja called after a week to clarify the situation. She distinctly remembered the conviction with which the doctor had decided to continue the higher dosage in light of the worsening weather.

"Why didn't the doctor factor in the scenario that the steroid-induced paranoia could be so severe?" Ninjja found herself still confused. "Was it an overcorrection for an expected problem, or just negligence? Or was it just the narrow focus on his own area of specialty?" She did not have an answer. Her father's scared face and nervousness had started gnawing at her. They asked the pulmonologist to have a word with the psychiatrist, with whom they were meeting next. Fortunately, he obliged.

It was getting difficult to keep her father focused and calm for the next appointment. He was so fidgety, nervous, and confused that he would make a request to head back home every couple of minutes. After a thirty-minute wait that seemed like an eternity, they were sitting face-to-face with the psychiatrist. After the first ten minutes, Ninjja's father started opening up and confessed to having severely negative thoughts. The psychiatrist explored the contours of the problem and then told the family that some antianxiety pills were a must at this stage.

Ninjja asked him to speak to the pulmonologist to align the two sets of treatments. Alas, he did not relish the thought of having to discuss his recommendation with another doctor. It became very obvious when he feigned that he was unable to get through to the other doctor.

Surprisingly, Ninjja's mother displayed unusual bravado by her standards and dialed the pulmonologist from her cell phone. Reluctantly, the two men had to speak. All that Ninjja could decipher was that the prescribed medicines were the mildest possible for the CNS (central nervous system) and that the dosage would be reduced in a week or so.

Once they were back home, Ninjja felt as though she were back from a battlefront. If only the doctors would work as a team!

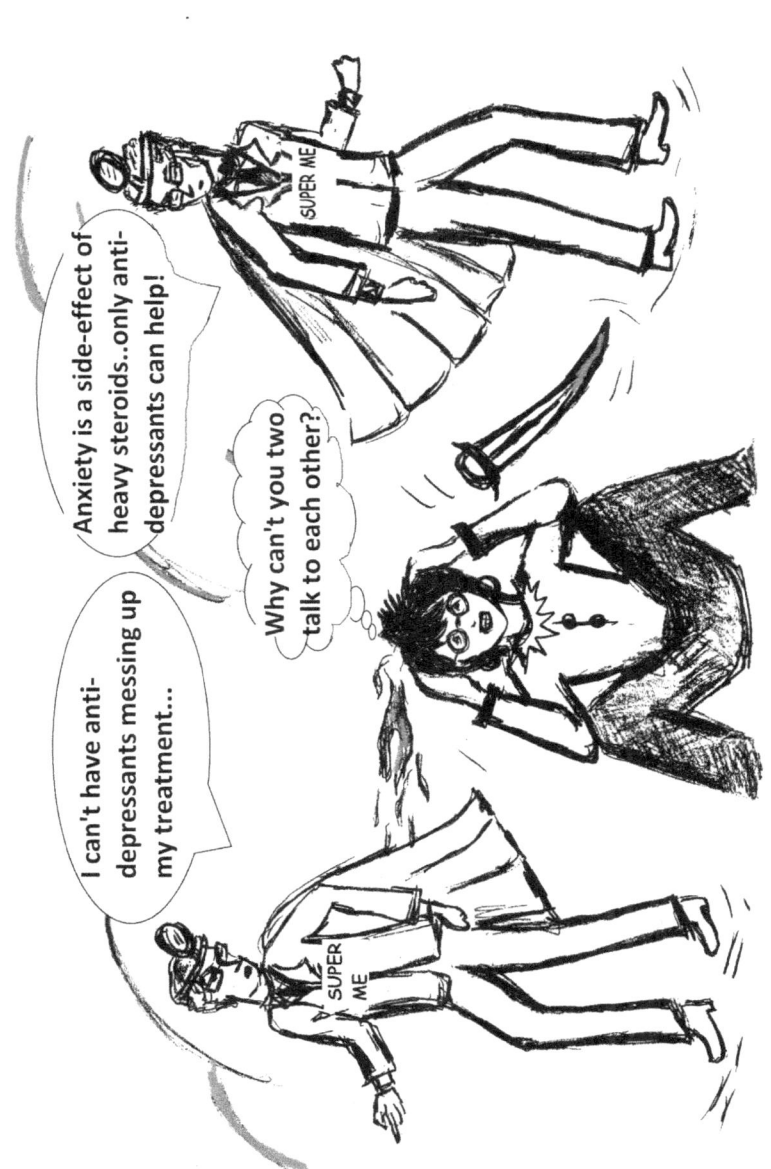

Ninja caught between two "SuperMeDocs"

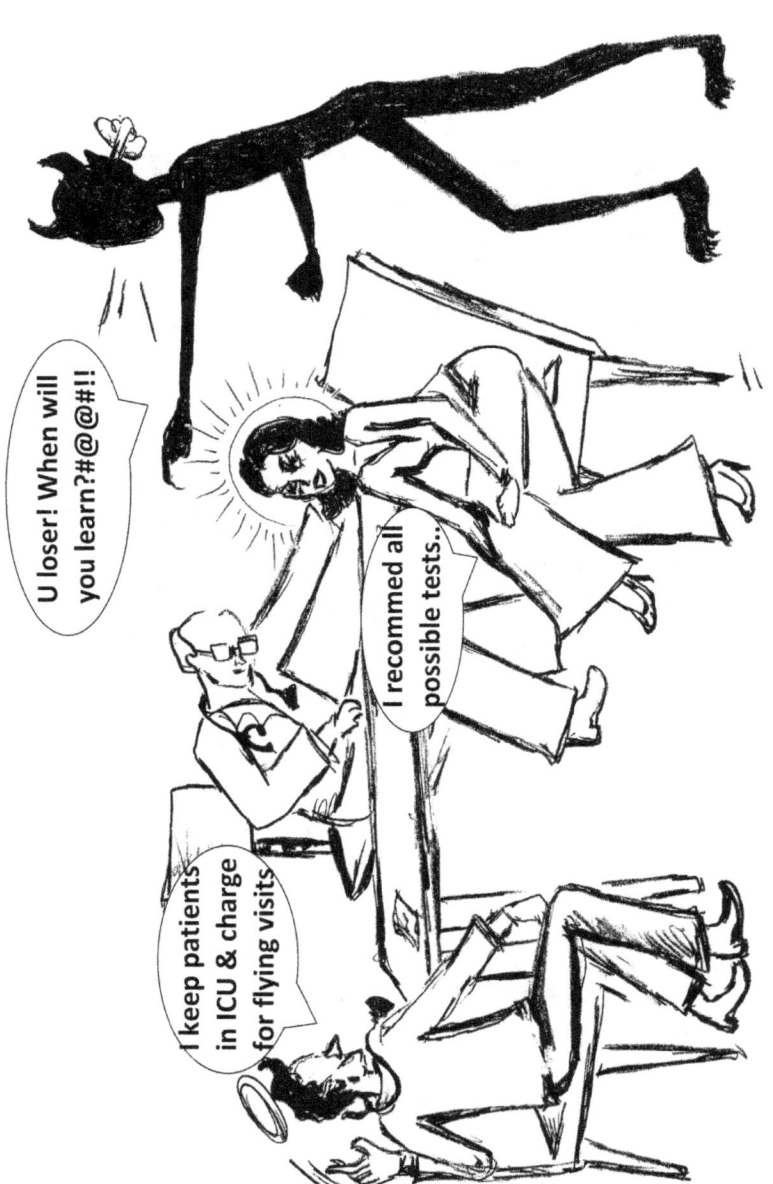

Ninjja's interpretation of performance review of remaining three categories of doctors

Eleven

The Tricky Balance

MARCH 2012

The combination of various treatments had started showing the right trajectory. Ninjja could see that continuous steroids coupled with multiple rounds of infections had made her father so fragile that the point of balance was becoming more and more precarious. The impact of any overdose was now magnified manifold. Ninjja vaguely remembered an analogous principle from her engineering training that complex systems had to be managed with precision control. It meant that the system's response had to be monitored at intervals of fractions of seconds, and smart corrective action had to be taken. The most advanced systems were intelligent enough to learn from previous experiences to adjust the control parameters for a better response.

Ninjja wondered if the advances in medical science would ever make it possible to manage the most complex machinery of the human body with such precision in the future. Even though this level of precision seemed fictional, Ninjja felt that it should not have been impossible for an experienced doctor to assess the symptoms of paranoia and psychosis during regular telephone conversations with the patient and his family and initiate a course correction.

Though Ninjja's father had taught her not to worry about things that were in the past (with his favorite Sanskrit saying of *"Gatam na shochyam"* [What is past must not be dwelled upon]), she couldn't get her mind off the suffering that her father had been going through over the past several weeks (and more so over the past year and a half). However hard she tried to pin it on destiny, she could not overlook the fact that a major source of his suffering still seemed man-made.

While the antianxiety pills were doing some work, Ninjja continued her attempts to get her father to talk about his anxieties and fears. He was very unlike his usual chatty self in this period and more so during such conversations. Ninjja had to piece together different tidbits to get a small glimpse of the scary cobweb that had been weaving itself in his head.

Ninjja was making her best efforts to disentangle him with scissors of logic and affection, when he finally spoke again: "When you talk like this, I can see the logic. I know that I am behaving oddly... but things just happen. I don't know why I suddenly panic, and I know that I am causing you all a lot of trouble," he said after a long pause.

Ninjja's heart skipped a beat, and her mother looked on in dismay. Ninjja's mother had been the 24-7 foot soldier on the battlefront with such intensity that the anxiety and stress were written all over her. She could probably do with some counseling herself, but instead she managed to find her inner resources to offer the right words of comfort.

That night, Ninjja went to bed feeling slightly relieved as she saw her father's inclination to talk about the problem as the first sign of recovery.

In a few days, Ninjja could see his mental state returning to normal, but the ordeal had taken a bigger toll on his physical condition. He found it hard to move around without any support. The ensemble of attendants was apparently only for cosmetic purposes. They found surfing TV channels and listening to music more befitting than responding to her father's feeble demands for help. Ninjja's harried mother had no energy left to control the unruly, shameless support staff that was being unleashed by the health-care agency. Finally, it took a full-blown blasting from Ninjja to propel them into some meaningful action. In her moments of frustration, she coined the term "DeafAndant" to describe these attendants who were deaf to the patient's voice.

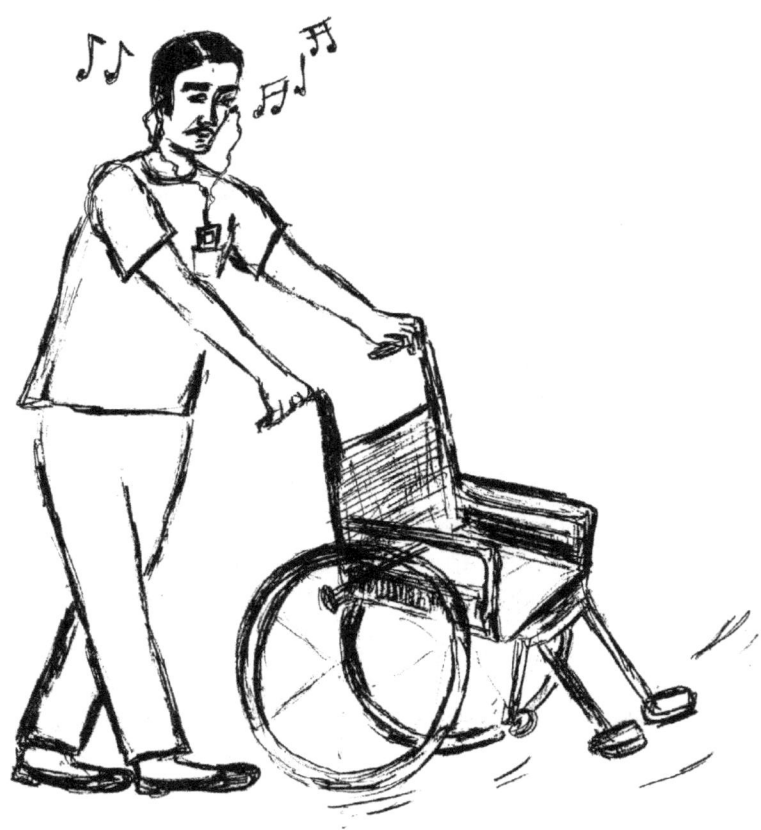

DeafAndant: Attendant...But is deaf to the patient's voice

Two weeks later, Ninjja was elated to find that her father had gone for a morning walk and did not need anyone to hold his hand. He was proudly holding his walking stick and declared that he did not need any support. In the sinusoidal journey that Ninjja had witnessed over the past two years, this was a sign of an uptick in the curve. Ninjja didn't want to pay attention to the fact that the amplitude as well as the frequency of such oscillations had been rising. She hoped and prayed for her father's state to stay on the upward curve this time and never turn the course.

The next day, despite her rush to get to work Ninjja couldn't help noticing that her father was looking somewhat grim. "Father, what happened? What are you thinking about?" she asked.

"Nothing, I am just a bit groggy." He shoved her away. Ninjja was well versed in his facial expressions by now and knew that this was beyond grogginess. She was getting late for work, so she made one last attempt at cheering him up: "Whatever it is, it is not worth thinking about. You were so cheerful yesterday. Bring back yesterday to today as well…and relax! I will talk to you in the evening."

Ninjja tasked her mother with finding out more and left in a hurry.

Later that evening, Ninjja was in for something unexpected.

"He has had a strange dream. That is what is worrying him," Ninjja's mother said in a hushed tone.

"A dream? That is hardly a reason to worry about. What was the dream about?"

"He wouldn't talk about it. It wasn't good is all that I have learned." Ninjja's mother looked concerned, and Ninjja was intrigued.

Ninjja sat beside her father and pretended that she was there to watch TV with him. After a long silence, she couldn't get herself to beat about the bush. She gently reached out for his hand and asked, "Father, why aren't you talking? Why are you thinking about the dream so much? You need to talk to us about it."

There was no response.

"You can tell us anything. You know how tough we are," Ninjja pleaded again.

"OK. I will tell you later," he said quietly, as though he wasn't comfortable speaking in her mother's presence. Ninjja's mother took the cue and moved away.

"What is it?" Ninjja looked at him with her wide, curious, bespectacled eyes.

"My time has come," he said slowly, squeezing her hand. Ninjja wasn't prepared for such an answer.

"What do you mean? How have you concluded this?"

"I saw yakshas [a form of nature spirit in Indian mythology]…it was dark, and it was raining," he said slowly. Ninjja could not believe what she was hearing, as was evident from her widened eyes and dropped jaw.

She recovered very quickly and challenged him. "This is your own fear showing up as a dream. This means nothing. Do you remember the dream I had once in school?" Ninjja continued her monologue: "I had seen a snake who wanted to bite me. Then, just at that very moment, the snake suddenly stopped and said, 'Oh! I was meant to come two years later,' and then disappeared. I thought I was going to die after two years and didn't tell you or Mother, lest you got anxious. But it had no meaning. Nothing happened after two years. Even after twenty years, I am still here. Are you listening to me?"

He bore a vacant expression. Finally, after a pause of a few minutes, she saw some movement.

"The dream came at the cusp of night and day...the yakshas that I saw were the bad ones...and the rain in darkness signifies something...in the distance, I also saw Yama [the god of death] himself... it is a sign!" he said, shaking his head, totally unfazed by Ninjja's reasoning.

Ninjja's heart almost stopped. She knew that her father was a believer in stars, signs, and the like. It was becoming increasingly clear that he had taken this strange dream to its deepest possible interpretation and had convinced himself of its veracity. She had no idea how to fight the demons from the other world. As the weapons of logic were failing, she resorted to using another one from the world of stars and signs itself to fight the battle on its home turf.

"Why don't you think of the jinx of seventy-five that you have just broken? Didn't you yourself say that the danger is over? Didn't the astrologer tell you that a golden period of your life has started?" Ninjja tried to field counterexamples so as to shake his belief. "And by the way, you cannot ignore the vital statistics. Your health is anything but declining. Someone needs to be totally out of his or her sensibilities to tell you something so crazy." She tried to laugh it off in her final attempt.

Ninjja's father gave a weak smile. His smile acknowledged Ninjja's sincere efforts, but his eyes still had something deep hidden in them. Ninjja was too keen to find any cues that suggested that her father was willing to put this behind him and embraced this as a first sign. Soon, he allowed her to change the topic of discussion and devolved to sharing his favorite jokes. Ninjja laughed the same way as she had when she had heard the joke for the first time in her childhood—about a hundred recitals ago.

. . .

Two days later, Ninjja's father had increased the pace and the distance of his morning walk and was demonstrating as many signs of good health as were possible in his condition.

He was eagerly awaiting her that evening. He could barely wait for her to remove her shoes and get a change of clothes.

"What happened?" Ninjja looked at him quizzically.

"I did a lot of important work today," he declared proudly. Ninjja's mother had a strange mix of amusement and concern written all over her face, and her father was doing his best to dramatize the event.

"Look what he has done!" she exclaimed, opening the door of the steel cupboard, which had become the repository of all the important documents over the years. For Ninjja, it was like a black hole that had a perennial appetite for paper. Ninjja glanced around to see if she could spot any difference from the last time she had visited this cupboard. It did not take very long for her to spot a fresh, white piece of paper that was neatly stuck behind one of the doors. It had her father's confident, neat handwriting.

"What is all this, Father?" Ninjja instinctively asked as she stepped forward to have a closer look. Thirty seconds of staring at the sheet obviated the need for any answers from her father's pursed lips.

"Well, well, well! You are too funny…and cute!" Ninjja remarked, trying to laugh off what she had just seen. "Shall we say that this is your will?" she continued, while her father looked on with a content smile.

"What was the need to write a letter addressed to me and my sister asking us to split whatever you leave behind in equal ratio? And that we should take good care of our mother? Isn't this obvious? And by the way, you are not going anywhere so soon!" Ninjja ended her sentence emphatically.

"Yes, I know that the two of you won't fight over money, but it is best to put everything in black and white," came an equally emphatic reply from her father.

By now Ninjja knew that the dream was far from being out of her father's life. It was clearly guiding a lot of his behavior. Ninjja tried to hide her concern and instead tried to trivialize the episode. "By the way, what makes you think that we are so mean that we won't take care of our mother unless it is expressed as your last wish?" Ninjja continued her monologue with a serious expression. "Also, I have no intention of sharing anything with my sister. Since you have made me a joint holder in all your accounts, I will empty them instantly and disappear."

She watched her father's expression change in a jiffy, and she burst out laughing. For a split second, her gullible father had fallen for her guile. He soon joined her in her laughter upon realizing that he had been caught. Ninjja's stern mother couldn't hold onto her stiff upper lip, either.

After dinner, Ninjja's father thought of explaining himself and easing the tension that he perceived in Ninjja.

"Please don't think that I am crazy. I am not worried about the dream, but at the same time, one needs to plan for these eventualities. It is the eternal truth...yet I am not ready to face it. I feel attached to you all. After I am gone, who will love you all the way I do? There is so much more left to do." He held Ninjja's hand between both his palms and looked at her affectionately.

Ninjja was moved to see this real tussle between philosophy and reality. It was her father who had taught her young mind the concepts of maya (illusion), karma, shoonya (zero), poornam (whole), and anant (infinity) from ancient Indian scriptures. Even after growing up, Ninjja used to find it hard to fully appreciate the concepts individually, and the deeper interlinkages used to fox her even more. Having looked up to her father as the guru who would enlighten her, she couldn't watch him struggle with the blurring line between the real and the esoteric.

However, the next moment she found herself questioning her own thinking: *Who am I to decide what is indeed real? Maybe I am just looking at one state of reality that I am capable of seeing.* A lot of things she had heard all her life from her father came together, and she suddenly found her voice:

"Father, didn't you tell me that everything is part of infinity? There is nothing like an end...we move on a continuum...do you remember? Then why are you thinking about the end? Everything around us could be maya—isn't it? Then why worry about leaving behind something that wasn't real to begin with? Again, leaving behind doesn't mean anything, as one might be just moving from one state to the other. This feeling of emptiness or shoonya that is engulfing you is also part of infinity." Ninjja paused for a breath and noticed that her father was staring at her with love and pride. His peaceful, blue eyes had a shine in them.

She felt encouraged and continued, "Didn't you tell me that all we need to focus on is karma in this life? And that's what you have always done...so why think about something over which no one has any control? I am going to repeat your favorite statement now—'There are three unknowns about death: when, where, and how.' So just let it be...and focus on enjoying today." Ninjja stopped and squeezed her father's hand to reassure him. He was now smiling. He ran his hand affectionately over her head in a gesture of appreciation and blessing. He looked pleased to hear the spirit of his own thinking through his daughter's mouth.

Ninjja now found her father at peace with himself. She was now convinced that her father was an evolved being to have even articulated his dilemma. It did not take him very long to take a pragmatic perspective of the dark issues that were bothering him. Soon they were back to current reality and found themselves engrossed in watching his favorite TV program.

During the drive to work, Ninjja felt like calling Arv. Fortunately, he spared her his usual sarcasm and told her another recent story of his near escape from an arranged marriage.

"Unfortunately, despite my best efforts, I was taken to the second round this time…and the girl was just perfect! One hundred percent true to the parameters of my parents," he added later. Ninjja knew that she wouldn't need to push him to get to his reasoning. "But I chickened out. Come to think of it—spending your life with a perfect stranger that is a product of a mathematical equation? I can't do this. I would be happier with someone who is not actually perfect…but someone whom I can laugh with, share my inner thoughts without the fear of being judged…and just be myself and let the other person be…" he continued.

Ninjja couldn't agree more, but she chose to remain silent for fear of thrusting Arv toward permanent bachelorhood.

Finally, Arv enquired about her father's health and ended on a note that was very unlike him: "Ninjja, I am glad that you called. I was missing you…bye, till we meet again." There was something that touched a chord in her heart. She was quick to dismiss it as a passing thought and moved on to fight the twister that was awaiting her at work.

· · ·

MAY 2012

On the home front, things had returned to as normal as they could be. A full-time houseboy whom Ninjja had found from a friend's village was marvelous. In no time, he had taken on more responsibilities than Ninjja could have ever hoped for. Ninjja's parents had been extremely apprehensive, considering the innumerable news stories of crimes committed by domestic help. However, Ninjja's due diligence had given her the comfort to overrule them and implant him with her parents.

In no time, he had won over the hearts of both of them, which was no mean feat to achieve. The time required for Ninjja to manage the daily home affairs had dropped dramatically. More importantly, she was happier that some positive energy awaited her at home in the evening instead of the regular tension.

One afternoon Ninjja was pleasantly surprised to find her father happily engaged in a game of chess with this new personality in their home. "I am impressed," she exclaimed. "I think I am ready to declare you fully fit and fine."

Ninjja's father had a beaming smile and chirped, "I was going to tell you the same. Let's plan to go out somewhere."

"Done! There is a new, undulating highway…one gets fascinating skyline views of the city. I will take you for a drive at night. We can even eat out if you feel up to it. There is a very nice, exclusive restaurant, and if we go early enough, it will feel like our own private one!" Ninjja said encouragingly. She did not want to take any risks with visiting crowded places again.

Unfortunately, an unannounced visitor, a schedule change from the physiotherapist, and a never-ending meeting Ninjja got stuck in, were a few of the many reasons that got in the way of realizing this short, sweet trip for a couple of days.

"Father, come what may, we shall definitely go tomorrow. Let us all take this as sacrosanct now," Ninjja reassured her father in a determined way that evening.

Ninjja started her work really early in the hope of freeing up the evening to fulfill the promise she had made to her father. She was all excited to announce her arrival well before six o'clock and couldn't wait to be in her father's room. To her surprise, he did not share her excitement. He was looking tired, despite his best attempt to smile.

"He has a mild stomach pain and fever," Ninjja's mother responded to Ninjja's quizzical eyes.

"Oh, in that case, you need to rest," Ninjja said in a comforting tone. Ninjja wasn't pleased with this new impediment, but she wasn't overly worried either, as the stomach had been a weak spot for her father ever since she could remember. After hearing the symptoms, she advised him to take the usual herbal medicine that had proven its effectiveness time and again. In the meanwhile, Ninjja's mother had already spoken to the doctor and had started a course of antibiotics, lest the fever be a symptom of something more vicious.

The next morning, the fever had subsided, but her father continued to complain about his stomach. "It must be gas," everyone said, including the doctor. Some additional antacids were prescribed, and the lack of relief was construed to be a combination of time needed for medicines to act and her father's habit of exaggeration of the real magnitude of problem.

Ninjja wasn't very concerned, as her father's condition didn't look any different than a minor vibration in an undulating graph (which had become the new steady state).

•   •   •

Around eleven in the morning, Ninjja's phone rang. She was deeply engrossed in her work and saw the phone as an irritant. She hoped that the caller would hang up after a couple of rings. However, the ringing continued. Ninjja noticed her father's name and picked up the phone reluctantly. "Yes, Father, what is it?"

"Bol, Beta [speak, my dear child]," said an affectionate voice on the other end. The same exchange continued for couple of rounds, frustrating Ninjja somewhat.

"Father, you have called. You need to tell me why you have called me at work. Is there anything urgent?" Her tone bore minor tinges of irritation.

"No, Beta, you have called. I was actually sleeping, and the attendant brought the phone to me," he continued in the same affectionate tone.

At least there was an explanation now of the awkward initial conversation. Ninjja still couldn't understand how the phone could have been ringing at both ends. She decided not to spend any more time on unraveling this telecommunication marvel and asked her father to go back to taking rest. She tried to refocus her attention to work that did not come easily.

Ninjja had started her day before sunrise, and now, well past sunset, she was headed to the airport. This was another usual workday when she was deprived of witnessing the fundamental phenomena of the universe (sunrise and sunset) that her human ancestors so doggedly used as pegs to govern their lives. She realized that her father hadn't called her even in the evening. She felt a tad guilty for having ignored him. His affectionate voice during the morning chance call was still ringing in her head as she dialed her home phone.

• • •

Her father was sleeping. She also learned that the doctor's visit didn't materialize due to huge reluctance from her father, which was nothing unusual. Such things added to Ninjja's frustration, as there was only finite time available. She would have liked for some minor tasks to be done without her interference.

"But I did speak to the doctor...he has suggested another medicine for immediate relief." Ninjja's mother offered a lame defense.

"But the fact remains that he is still suffering from pain and is now almost on a liquid diet. It would have been better if the doctor had physically seen him. Forget it, I will take him tomorrow." Ninjja put the phone down with a mix of anger and frustration. To Ninjja, the situation was important enough to merit a visit to the doctor, but not critical enough to be a 'time sink' for her. She knew that her parents would never understand this distinction, yet her patience was running out.

The following day, Ninjja was concerned to see the level of distention in her father's stomach. Though he had been heavily endowed with a potbelly most of his life, this looked unusual.

• • •

After going through the usual rituals of coaxing, counseling, and cajoling Ninjja managed to get him to the hospital just in time for the doctor's appointment. She felt that her father's confidence was increasing as the distance from the hospital decreased. Having one's own wheelchair definitely saved some waiting time in forty-two degrees Celsius at the hospital gate.

The doctor's assistant had formed a special bond with her father and always went out of her way to make him comfortable. Unfortunately, the doctor couldn't keep his promised appointment. Fifteen minutes turned to half an hour and soon into one and a half hours. The assistant apologized profusely, claiming that the doctor was stuck with an emergency case in the ICU. Like everything else, the concepts of pain and criticality are also relative. Yet Ninjja was unable to keep her mind off the distress that was visible in her father's eyes, despite his best efforts to hide his true state.

Finally, they received the summons to show up in the emergency room for a thorough examination. It was some task to get her father to lie down on the emergency-room bed. His agony was now showing up in the form of groans with every small movement.

Upon examination, the doctor considered it a case of bloating due to excessive gas. He conducted a small procedure to provide immediate relief, prescribed some S.O.S. (medical abbreviation for 'if needed') medicines, and suggested that the antibiotics be stopped.

Ninjja asked a few follow-up questions, checked if any further tests were needed, and was told not to worry about it. She had a fleeting thought of the need to consult a gastro specialist. However, given the complication of the respiratory issues, she did not want to do anything without the consent of the pulmonologist.

•   •   •

While she had hoped to get back to work in the afternoon, the hospital visit ate away almost the whole day. She hoped for a better tomorrow, considered the day well spent, and started bracing up for a late night to make her deadlines.

The following day, there was no improvement in her father's health, and the discomfort continued. Given his recent history of taking a long time to heal from even a small blister, Ninjja considered time as the only dimension that had to now play out, considering everything else had been checked off.

The week was flying by. It was already Friday, and Ninjja was now getting concerned. She didn't think it would be practical to take him for another visit to the doctor. She was feeling trapped. Next, she tried her regular general physician, but he was out of the country. She was desperate for any doctor to come and have a look at her father, so she called a doctor in a small hospital next door and urged him to make a five-minute detour to visit her home. She even offered to pick him up if that was more convenient. Unfortunately, her plea went unanswered. The doctor was outright rude and hung up the phone on her.

Ninjja's strong determination had started cracking.

Her father's attending pulmonologist was not reachable. All the doors seemed to be closing on Ninjja.

•　•　•

On the following day, she managed to reach the pulmonologist around eleven in the morning after repeated attempts. He mentioned he was caught up in taking viva of medical students.

Ninjja apologized for disturbing him and went on, "There is no change in my father's bloated stomach or in his feeling of discomfort. He also had some fever last night...I am getting concerned, Doctor."

The doctor, who was probably used to constantly complaining patients, remained unmoved. "It will settle down. There is a common stomach flu these days. It will go away. We should just probably resume the antibiotic that we had stopped."

"But, Doctor, given that it has been almost a week now, and there is absolutely no improvement in the condition, do you want me to get any tests done?" Ninjja questioned him further, hesitantly.

The doctor paused for few seconds and replied, "Well, I don't see the need...but if you want to...then go ahead and do some of the basic tests—hemoglobin, RBC, WBC, etcetera." Ninjja hastily started scribbling on her palm, cursing herself for not being ready with a notepad.

She immediately relayed the message to her mother and asked her to make the necessary arrangements. Ninjja was glad that the service of sample collection from home was at least available for a fee. However, Ninjja was met with an unexpected response. Her mother was so fatigued, both mentally and physically, that she refused to call the clinic. "If the doctor hasn't insisted on the tests, then let it be...I won't call any more people," Ninjja's mother replied in an exhausted tone.

It was difficult for the family to understand the distinction between real issues and the exaggerated ones. Equally, it was hard to assess the severity and criticality of different ailments that had afflicted Ninjja's father from time to time. The reality was so blurred that it had started clouding the judgment of those who were expected to be in charge. Ninjja transmitted the same emotion back: "Fine. Suit yourself. I think it would be better to be doubly sure with tests. You can make your call. If you decide to call the laboratory, please request for getting the results back by tomorrow morning. Let's be clear: this time, I am definitely not calling them." Ninjja was curt in her response. One thing led to another, and soon enough, the exhaustion and curtness converted into a heated exchange.

Ninjja's father, who had been listening painfully for the past several minutes, gathered his leftover energy and wailed, "Oh! I feel miserable. All of this is happening because of me. I am causing you all so much trouble!" It was enough to get both women back to their senses. Within seconds, Ninjja was hugging her father and consoling him. She felt terrible for losing her cool when her father was in so much pain. Her mother dutifully resumed the task of calling up the laboratory.

Late afternoon soon turned into evening and then hid itself beneath the black curtain of night.

Ninjja's father was able to barely sleep, and Ninjja's mother kept the night vigil. There was nothing that they could do. All the prescribed medicines, including SOS for pain and several home remedies, had been tried.

The only option that was left was to take him to emergency, where the attending doctors would have no qualms about putting him into the ICU—a place of no return, at least in his current state.

Ninjja was petrified at even the thought of putting her father through this. Every time she asked him if he wanted to get admitted to the hospital, he shook his head vehemently, as though the experience of his previous confinement almost nineteen months ago was still fresh in his memory. He wasn't talking much, but whenever he spoke, he said that he didn't want to get admitted.

Ninjja knew that, given that this was the weekend, his regular physician would not show up until Monday. The idea of someone totally unfamiliar treating him, with her father's complex history, did not inspire any confidence.

Even if I were to give them a full file, how will they know his typical responsiveness to different medications? Experience has made us better at handling the increments in which steroids have to be tinkered with. How about interaction between different medicines? Ninjja remembered how paranoid the pulmonologist used to be if another doctor prescribed any new drug. *Will the new doctors learn from their experimentation at such a critical moment? How can they treat someone by just looking at current data without any context? What if they conduct more invasive tests? That would surely be the last nail in his weak system!* Ninjja found herself caught in a web with no visible exit.

Given that the probability of success looked even smaller in the alternative that Ninjja had just visualized, she decided to wait till the test results came through.

· · ·

The clinic started its operations in the mood of a lazy Sunday. The results that were supposed to come through in the morning actually arrived late afternoon. In the meanwhile, Ninjja's father continued to suffer silently. He kept lying on his bed most of the day with almost no appetite.

As Ninjja started looking through the test results, even her medically uneducated mind started seeing red flags everywhere.

The test results were way out of range on every parameter. *There must be some infection for sure.* Ninjja had a worried look. She didn't know if it would be sensible to share this information with her parents at this stage. She decided to call the doctor instead. Sunday is not a day when the doctors are most responsive to phone calls from patients, but fortunately, the pulmonologist picked up the phone.

A concerned Ninjja rattled out the results without any pause. The only reaction that she could hear from the doctor was an occasional "Oh." Given the pause at the other end, Ninjja wasn't sure if he had fully absorbed what she was saying.

"Looks like there is some infection, Doctor, doesn't it?" Ninjja tried to fill in the uncomfortable silence.

"Yes, it seems so," the doctor replied calmly.

"So what should we do?" Ninjja asked eagerly.

"We need to increase the dosage of the antibiotic," came the reply.

"Anything else?" Ninjja didn't feel comfortable with the answer.

The doctor just increased the dosage and then suggested that they meet on the coming day. Another minor procedure (an enema) was suggested to relieve the discomfort that had been harrowing her father. While the procedure was known to be so simple that people were able to do self-administration, Ninjja didn't want to take any chances. The attendant vouched for his experience with the procedure and offered to administer it. Yet Ninjja's risk aversion forced her to try very hard to get one of the hospital's senior nursing staff to visit.

· · ·

Ninjja's father was waiting expectantly. His eyes had a lot of hope, as though the visiting nurse were going to relieve him of his agony with a magic wand. His ever-positive attitude was giving him strength to calmly handle his discomfort. Ninjja saw this as another health hiccup that was taking much longer than needed.

The dark night went by, and Ninjja's mother didn't sleep a wink. She didn't want to disturb Ninjja's sleep for fear of upsetting her Monday-morning schedule.

Around five in the morning, when she was pulled in, her father was not looking too good. He was groaning in pain with his eyes closed. He looked half asleep and was not very responsive to questions. Ninjja was swinging between concern and helplessness. After offering water to his parched lips, Ninjja started desperately waiting for eight o'clock so that she could call the doctor.

Twelve

The Ultimate Verdict

The doctor listened but was unmoved. Ninjja made a desperate plea to him to visit her home. However, the doctor's demeanor was in exact contrast to the turmoil that Ninjja was feeling. He asked her to call in the ambulance and bring her father to the hospital. He assured her that she shouldn't worry and that this would be the best course of action. It was a scary thought, but there didn't seem any option.

With a heavy heart, Ninjja picked up the phone to call the ambulance.

The normally unconcerned attendant, who had been watching the misery for so long, finally spoke. "You have been taking care of your father so gently. The ambulance guys are ruthless...I see them every day. They will treat him like a piece of luggage and deliver him to the hospital. Why do you want to do that? Why don't you take him in your car? It is a pretty big one...he will be comfortable."

He sounded compassionate and genuine. Ninjja was touched by his gesture and cut the call that she had dialed. She ran inside to get her father ready for the hospital.

• • •

Ninjja's mother looked so lost that she was going about her regular chores without any concern for the most critical step at that point. Through the night, her father's responsiveness had become much worse, yet Ninjja was able to get enough response to get him to clean up, change, and get seated in the wheelchair with the help of the attendant. Her father was responding through nods with his eyes closed. At that moment, the phone rang.

Ninjja's sister was at the other end. She had been running a very tight schedule for the past week and hadn't had the time to call. Ninjja picked up the phone and put her on speaker for her father to listen. However, there was no change in his disposition. He continued his rhythmic groaning.

Ninjja's sister was in for a deep shock. Just a week ago, she had chatted with him for hours, where he had been so cheerful…and now, she couldn't even hear a coherent word! Ninjja realized her mistake and grabbed the phone.

"Don't you worry. He has become very weak due to a stomach problem since last week. We are taking him to the hospital. You should be able to speak to him tomorrow. I will call you later." Ninjja wanted to assuage her concern as well as get moving quickly toward the hospital.

It was getting more difficult with every passing moment. She was numbed to see that her father's behavior was close to that of someone who was unconscious. Ninjja ran back to get a bunch of pillows to make him comfortable. She instructed the attendant and the domestic help to keep a close watch on her father and make sure he didn't get hurt during their upcoming encounter with the multitude of bumps and potholes on the road. She had never jumped into the driver's seat feeling so out of synch with her surroundings before.

The reception at the emergency door of the hospital was nothing unusual. In no time, Ninjja's father was pulled out like a piece of luggage and deposited on a bed. The staff sprang into action.

Ninjja and her mother were watching with blank eyes. At this stage, there was nothing that they could do or say. Soon they were asked to leave the emergency room and wait outside.

Within ten minutes, the pulmonologist arrived. After two minutes of discussion with the emergency-room doctors and one glance at her father, he pronounced, "To me it looks like a septic shock. He is dying."

The last word reverberated in Ninjja's ears with such intensity that it felt like her eardrums would explode.

There must have been some mistake. Ninjja's inner voice was talking to her now. *How can this be? Four days back, he was dismissed from this hospital by this very doctor saying that it was a minor issue...just eighteen hours ago, when I called up the doctor with the test results, he did not raise any alarm...and now...such a drastic pronouncement!* She continued talking to herself. Her voice was stuck in her throat.

With this pronouncement, the doctor did walk up to her mother to tell her to have courage. He told her that they would try to do whatever was medically possible at this stage. He also advised her that if the situation ever came to using a ventilator or artificial resuscitation, then the family should refrain from it.

However, at this stage, the doctor's supposed gesture of concern and kindness toward the family did not touch any corner of Ninjja's heart.

The situation had gone dramatically opposite to what Ninjja had imagined. She tried to console her mother, who seemed to have lost her power to react. The attendant and the domestic help had tears in their eyes. Ninjja's emotions were bottled up so tightly that she started going about the mundane activities like a robot: swiping her credit card for the ICU admission and filling out forms.

An hour had passed by, and she hadn't seen her father yet. He was still lost in transit between the emergency room and the ICU. It suddenly struck Ninjja that it was time to call her sister!

She mustered all her courage to speak the words she had never imagined she would have to: "You need to take the next flight and come down here…he is probably going."

Ninjja didn't know how the last few words left her mouth. The long silence at the other end told her that it was even more difficult for the person who was listening.

"I…am…on my way!" Ninjja's sister finally spoke. The pause and broken words were a reflection of the emotional avalanche that she was caught in. Thousands of miles separated them, but they were still united in their grief. Not many words were spoken, but they could still feel each other's internal turbulence. The bond of silence had become all-encompassing when the nurse interrupted Ninjja.

"You can now move to the ICU. Your father has been transferred there."

Ninjja eagerly collected her dazed mother and moved as fast as she could to see her father. Unfortunately, the nurse's message was not supposed to be interpreted as a signal to meet her father but instead implied that now the waiting area had shifted. The long wait and lack of information was to continue for few more hours. Another Amazonian guard was at the ICU door. She was using the strength of her rough language and steely eyes to turn away the bewildered relatives of people who were incarcerated in the ICU. Sharing information and being kind had absolutely no position in her job description. Ninjja had a sense of déjà vu.

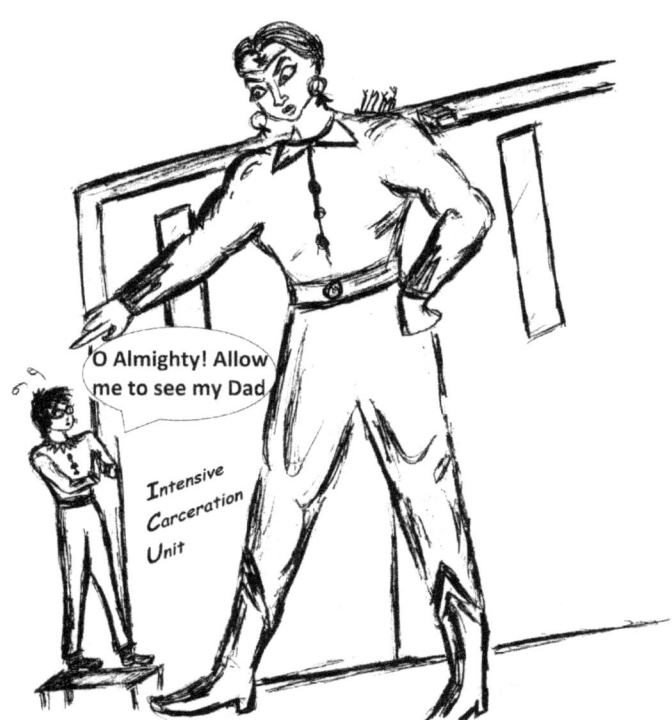

Ninjja pleading with Guardazonian

Ninjja's jitters were broken by a loud argument between the guard and a distraught relative. "How can you tell me to be patient? It has been twelve hours since I brought my mother here, and I have no news! What is going on? Is this a joke?" The man had totally lost his cool, and even a softening stance from the scare-mongering guard could not calm him down.

Twelve hours! Did I hear it right, or am I losing my mind? Ninjja tried to follow the conversation closely and reconfirmed that what she had heard was right. Ninjja was glad that her mother hadn't heard this unbelievable situation of someone being kept in the dark for twelve hours about the condition of a near and dear one. Finally, a medical supervisor and a doctor came forward to share some information with the haggard man. Ninjja was watching sympathetically and hoped that there was some good news awaiting him. At the same time, this precedent was shouting out loud that Ninjja needed to take some swift action if she wanted to see her father soon. She remembered a friend who had a relative in the administration department. Since the normal processes didn't seem to function, Ninjja decided to call in a favor.

Sure enough, thirty minutes later, she was allowed to enter the ICU and look at her father, who seemed to be in a deep sleep. Ninjja squeezed his hand, and she could feel that he was trying to respond with a small movement of his eyeballs. The sheer number of needles pricked in his body that were attached to various drips was enough to cause a piercing pain in Ninjja's heart. She hoped that all of this was being done with the good intention of making her father get better.

• • •

She was called in again to sign some papers. These documents were meant to reconfirm that the family did not want the patient to be put on a ventilator or use any other artificial resuscitation methods. One glance at the title of the document—"End of Life Agreement"—was enough to cause gut-wrenching pain. She somehow went through the signing process and walked out as fast as she could.

Ninjja resumed her sitting position next to her mother, tilted her head to the side, closed her eyes, and pretended to sleep to avoid a difficult conversation.

Fortunately, one of the neighbors dropped by and forced them to carry on with essential chores of life—like eating. In their present state of mind, they could have been fed with ash instead of delectable food, and they wouldn't have known.

However, the food did play a role in reigniting Ninjja's numbed brain, and she started replaying the events of the past four or five days in front of her closed eyes. The stark change in the doctor's proclamation came back to bite her. Going from a declaration of "Nothing serious...this is a normal stomach flu that is going around" to the confident statement of "This is septic shock...he is dying" felt too appalling. The words kept hammering in her head like a wild sea wave. She didn't know if there was something that she could do at this stage other than just pray. She stepped out for some fresh air and found herself dialing Uma's number in the hope of finding some solace. Uma was out of town. She consoled her and offered her some philosophical perspectives about life and death that, at best, served as the support of a floating branch to a sinking ship.

Next she dialed Arv. His reaction was more like a normal human, as he expressed shock and dismay. He offered her hope: "I think the doctor has taken an extreme position so that you are prepared for the worst. After setting expectations for such a desperate outcome, anything that happens will be a positive. So just chill! I think your father will come out of this, just the way he has done it on many previous occasions. It seems difficult to imagine that the situation could have tumbled down so dramatically within a span of a few days under the watchful eyes of the same doctor…was this great doctor sleeping all through it?" Now the anger was evident in Arv's voice. "You just hang in there. I will be back tomorrow, and I will be there with you as soon as I can." He tried to sound as positive as he could under the circumstances.

Ninjja realized that talking to her close circle was giving her more courage to handle the situation. Next she called up Raj and few of the close relatives, who were all saddened to hear the news but told her to have courage. Unfortunately, no one was in a position to physically be with her in this trying time.

· · ·

Ninjja realized that her mother was probably all by herself and, in her numbed state, needed her more than anything else.

· · ·

There was an announcement! A terrible pronunciation accompanied by an ear-piercing voice made it difficult to decipher what was being said. After straining her eardrums, along with some skillful interpretation of the distorted words that were being jettisoned, Ninjja realized that the Amazonian woman was calling out for relatives and attendants of her father!

"Oh, my God! It's for us!" Ninjja immediately sprang up from her chair and scurried toward the heavily guarded door. The next two minutes were full of anxiety, as she was told nothing while being ush-ered toward her father's bed. Ninjja was sprinting, with her mother trying her best to push her weak knees faster. Ninjja was filled with mixed emotions as she saw her father—happiness as well as pain.

Her father had regained consciousness but was not able to speak due to a tightly fitted oxygen mask. With all his energy, he lifted both his hands and gestured to Ninjja to come closer to him. Within seconds, he was flanked by Ninjja and her mother on either side. Ninjja grabbed his arm and put it around her. She could see tears trickling down his cheeks. He was shaking his head to communicate, as the tightly fastened mask had robbed him of his ability to speak. The ruthlessness with which it was installed was appalling. One side of the strap had partially covered an eye, and the other side had twisted his ear. Ninjja wondered if the staff considered ICU patients objects of experimentation or considered them human beings who actually did feel pleasure and pain!

Instead of being extra careful with the patient, who was unable to communicate his discomforts, they were taking advantage of the situation. "Be callous with patients who can't protest" seemed to be the motto. Because, for the foreseeable future, there was no option but to be at the mercy of these guardian angels, Ninjja controlled her anger and requested more careful handling. She hoped that her subtle way of showing the evidence of multiple examples of callous-ness would instill some shame, a critical precursor for behavioral change.

Unfortunately, the nursing staff did not permit them to remove the mask, eliminating all possibility of verbal communication. All they could do was to say a few comforting words and stroke his head.

His tears of helplessness were too overwhelming for Ninjja to look at. She wiped them off surreptitiously, hoping that she could create the illusion of their nonexistence. Both mother and daughter tried to put forward their guesses on what he was trying to say, but he vehemently shook his head, denying them the satisfaction of guessing his mind. Before they could try any further, the nurse gave them the signal to leave. Ninjja decided to ignore the signal and continued her one-way dialogue. However, she had underestimated the guardian angels! They were made of a much tougher material that was bolstered with a Teflon coating: nothing could permeate, and nothing could stick!

The nurse walked up to her and ordered her to leave. Earnest gestures from her father that clearly indicated that he wanted her to stay did not have any impact on the nurse's decision.

"Father, they are saying that the visiting time is up. We need to go," Ninjja whispered to her father with a heavy heart. He shook his head in protest and lifted his hand, telling her to stay. Ninjja was pained. What was the logic of keeping a man away from his family when a declaration of his impending death was already made? Ninjja was feeling horribly trapped. It occurred to her that health-care was the only business in the world where the customer's opinion didn't matter! Customers had to still beg for the mercy of the care providers, despite emptying their pockets and all the foreseeable reserves! *Probably, that's why this business never uses the term "customer"!*

Ninjja and her mother stepped back into the waiting area with hearts burdened, as if with a bag full of stones. All they wanted to do was to communicate with their ailing loved one. Ninjja knew that once they were thrown out, it would be nearly impossible to even get any information regarding the patient's condition. The notice board that said that the waiting relatives could call a certain number to inquire was nothing but a sham. The odds of getting the call answered were one in twenty, and then the probability of getting someone to respond with compassion was even smaller.

Why can't the health-care system use technology to lessen some of this pain? Would it be so hard to set up viewing screens in the outside area with appropriate passwords and controls so that individuals could watch their loved ones, at least from outside, and view the vitals instead of having to beg with the ICU staff to share the information? Ninjja was debating with herself. Her skeptic alter ego tried to raise questions about the feasibility. *I am sure the doctors don't want the family to watch while certain procedures are being performed. It may not be desirable, either!* Ninjja tried to argue back. *I understand that. That's why I suggested appropriate control mechanisms. I am sure it would not be very hard to switch off the viewing camera when needed.*

Ninjja continued her soliloquy. *I am not a technology expert, but based on what little I know, if some experts were to apply their minds to this challenge, a simple and cost-effective solution could be found.*

Ninjja closed her eyes in the hope of finding some solace.

· · ·

Her befuddled mind came back to consciousness with the sound of loud music, as a fellow waiting person had decided to turn up the TV to the maximum decibel level allowable by the system. It was strange to see such a colossal disregard for courtesy toward the other poor souls in the waiting area.

Despite the fact that Ninjja had lost part of her hearing during a childhood prank played by a friend, the impact of the loudness on her tired brain was like a team of heavyweight champions jumping on a percussion instrument. Ninjja's attempt to save herself by using a pillow as an ear muffler was worthless. She looked at the Amazonian guard at the door expectantly to step in with her rulebook, but there was no movement on that front. It did look like she was concerned only with protecting the door with all her might, and whatever happened at either side of the door was the least of her consideration.

Ninjja was in no mood to provide courtesy lessons to the potentially impervious rock sitting next to her, so she picked up her belongings, shook her mother from her dazed state, and moved to a corner at the far end of the hall. Fortunately, most of the people in that area were sleeping, reducing the risk of any sonic shock.

Once the status quo was resumed, the grief struck back with even more powerful stinging claws. "I hope he has gone back to sleep," Ninjja said to her mother hopelessly. "At least he will be spared the pain of being kept away from his family." Her voice trailed off.

A couple of hours later, it was time for the doctor's regular night round, and fortunately, Ninjja was called inside to witness the doctor's review. Ninjja saw that a group of young doctors was assembled around the senior doctor, and they were rattling off various medical parameters. "We don't see any hope" was what Ninjja heard from a distance with a sinking heart. The senior doctor then pulled out the logbook and started explaining several other indicators that were showing positive movement. He suggested certain changes to the medication and asked the team to keep up hope. "Oh, you are here!" he exclaimed as Ninjja approached. "The good news is that he is responding to medication. We will keep trying and hope for the best." He provided a positive vibe for the first time since Ninjja had set foot inside the hospital.

"Thank you, Doctor, for the uplifting talk that you gave to your team...because if they give up, I don't see what else will work."

"No...no, they won't give up. They will keep doing their best."

Ninjja cast a loving glance at her father before continuing her conversation. Later, she stole few moments to stroke her father's forehead and adjust his blanket.

In contrast to the scorching sun of tropical May, the air conditioner was running at the temperature of Arctic summer. The blanket was loosely covering the lower half of his body, and the upper half was at the mercy of the blue hospital robe that all the patients were wrapped in. "I am sure he is feeling cold. I am shivering myself," she called out to a nurse within audible distance and requested for another blanket. Her request was fulfilled quickly, but Ninjja didn't get the confidence that anyone inside would be concerned with worrying about small things like a patient's comfort with the ambient conditions! Without thinking much, she ran after the doctor who was near the exit door after completing his round.

"Doctor! I have a request. Why can't we continue the same treatment in a private room? At least he can be with his family...we can communicate whenever he wakes up," Ninjja pleaded but was summarily dismissed.

Soon, time dissolved into darkness, but there were no angels or fairies to add sparkle to Ninjja's bleak heart with their magical powers. Ninjja's mother managed to sneak in for five minutes to wish good-night to her husband—thanks to the grace of the new guard, the Almighty.

Both women huddled up in the reasonably comfortable waiting-room chairs and hoped for the best. They created a restful position for their bodies with the support of pillows.

Their brains were still unstoppable, though! They kept weaving many strange stories and scenarios that spanned the whole range of totally scary to completely optimistic.

As promised, Arv showed up at the hospital in the morning. He tried his best at a pep talk to bring some life back to their ashen faces.

The rest of the day went by, rocking between small rays of hope and complete despair. Arv proved to be the solid rock of support for the heavily undulating boat that Ninjja was riding in. Such a serious and responsible side of Arv was unknown to her even after knowing him for so long. It was a pleasant surprise that encouraged her to think about the many layers of human nature that remained unknown till the right trigger came along to expose them. She started hoping for a secret ingredient that was hidden in her father's immune system that could kick in now to fight the sepsis that was poisoning him.

· · ·

Ninjja was summoned inside hurriedly, as though something bad was happening. Ninjja was discovering new shades of "bad" as she went along. She learned in passing that the "patient had started throwing up his hands...and probably this was the end!"

Ninjja had never seen anyone die before and was sadly discovering such gruesome facts in case of her own father. She automatically joined her hands in prayer and asked God to have mercy. She was stopped from going near the bed as several doctors and nurses were surrounding her father and were doing something.

Soon after, she was told that he had been stabilized and that Ninjja could see him. It didn't feel like there had been such a crisis just few minutes ago. He was sleeping peacefully with his oxygen mask. Ninjja went near him and held his hand. As she ran her hand through his hair, she called out for him aloud. He opened his eyes for few seconds to look at her and then fell asleep again. Ninjja took this as a sign that he was probably semiconscious and thought that he might be able to hear her.

She went closer and whispered in his ear, "Baba, you have to have faith. Keep fighting…Sister is already on the flight. You have to see her." She repeated the same thing in different forms and tones a few times in the hope that something would get registered.

· · ·

Ninjja's sister arrived well past midnight. Due to the favors that Ninjja had called upon, fortunately she was allowed to see her father even in the official blackout hours. Ninjja couldn't fathom why a grief-stricken, anxious son or daughter who had flown for more than twenty-four hours to see a dying father had to take special favors to even see him.

Ninjja remembered the occasion when she had visited another famous hospital to see a friend's critically ill mother. The moment she had mentioned the name of the patient, entry and exit to the ICU had been extremely peaceful, with no constraints, except for the usual security checks and additional confirmation from the patient's family. At that time Ninjja hadn't attributed much significance to the VVIP status that her friend's family enjoyed. Now, contrasting that with her situation, the difference became stark. *Do VVIPs have much stronger emotions? Do they love their parents more? Why are their family members allowed to be with the patient in the ICU at all times, while the normal paying customers (as opposed to VVIPs, who are funded with taxpayers' money) have to be content with thirty-minute slots of two visiting hours or beg constantly?* Ninjja was overcome with mixed emotions of anger and grief.

This was the unwritten caste system that no one even thought of protesting against. The general acceptance of differential treatment (be it in the hospitals or on the roads or for any other public service) offered it the legitimacy of being propagated.

"At least in your country, the rules are the same for the rich and the poor…for the VVIPs and the commoners…if there are provisions for exceptions, I am sure they would be equally available for all," Ninjja blurted out to her sister. In return she got a confused look from someone who was clueless regarding the commotion going on in Ninjja's head about the prevalent inequality, even in moments of grief.

•   •   •

The status quo was maintained the next day. Ninjja's father regained consciousness momentarily, opened his eyes wide to recognize the presence of her sister, and nodded. It felt as soothing as a dewdrop on a parched tree.

Ninjja's sister was able to think more clearly in this time of despair and continued her endeavors to find a private room. Her persistence finally paid off.

"We will get him transferred to the private room, and then you can be with him. We will inform you," the junior doctor replied in a compassionate tone and sped away.

The family expectantly started waiting for the moment when they all could be in the same room at the same time. Soon, seconds turned into minutes and then into hours. The ICU gate remained fortified enough to not let any information out. As always, the telephone number that was supposed to share information went unanswered. After two hours of waiting, Ninjja was sufficiently aggravated to start creating noise in the system.

* * *

Finally, another hour later, they found themselves in the company of her father, who seemed to be in an even deeper sleep.

Whether three hours was the regular response time of the hospital to implement such a task or whether it was hurried by a few minutes or a few hours due to Ninjja's ruckus was hard to tell!

It was already past nine o'clock. Ninjja stepped out to relieve Arv, who had dropped by in the evening to check on her father. His presence had meant a lot to her, and her expression while saying good-bye probably gave it away.

There were unwritten rules for the private room as well, where they didn't want more than one attending person to sit. The objective was met by ensuring that only one chair was provided under any circumstances. Ninjja and her sister were undeterred and decided to share the chair and the armrest between them. They sent their mother out to the waiting area with a promise that they would call her if he woke up.

* * *

At two in the morning, Ninjja noticed some movement in her father's eyes…and then his hands. She shook her sister excitedly, who was half asleep due to mental exhaustion made worse by the jet lag. Within seconds they were at his side, calling out his name. He opened his eyes and looked at both of them with his full strength. He had to strain his eyes to absorb his whereabouts.

"Baba, can you hear us?" Ninjja's sister said loudly, squeezing his hand. After seeing his nod, there was no end to their delight. It seemed as though they had found the coveted pearl in the ocean. This was the first time that he was trying to say something with words, but due to the oxygen mask, one couldn't make out anything. Ninjja tried to read his lips and realized that he was calling out for her mother. Ninjja repeated whatever she had inferred and was elated to see him nod. This was the first time in over sixty hours that there was some communication going on. "Oh, she is right here…I will get her in a minute…hold on," Ninjja blurted and bolted out to get her mother.

After seeing his whole family, there was a sense of satisfaction in his eyes. Ninjja's sister noticed that the heavy swelling in his hands and legs that had been there earlier was gone. "Look here, Ninjja, his hands are looking normal now!" she shouted out in excitement.

Ninjja's father continued to say something, which they found difficult to decipher. After several guesses, they understood that he was talking about the oxygen mask, which was hurting his nose. Sure enough, on closer inspection, they realized that the mask was so tightly secured that it had created a wound on the top of the nose. "I am sure better-quality masks are available...shouldn't this damn thing be much softer?" Ninjja blurted out in anger while slipping in a small cotton swab on the bruised area.

"Probably they believe that patients don't feel any pain due to heavy medication...and they are not in a position to complain," Ninjja's sister whispered in her ear in anguish.

Ninjja's mother was intently looking at her husband and asking him if he had any pain or discomfort. He continued to talk through his mask. He was asking for something! Ninjja's mother figured it out instantly—"Water." This discovery sent a bolt of pain down their spines.

"Oh, God! How come it didn't strike us earlier...it has been over sixty hours, and he has been submerged under this mask...without a single drop of water!" Ninjja's sister ran out to get the attending nurse.

He heard the concern and replied calmly, "But I am not allowed to remove the mask...also, he won't be able to swallow water due to these tubes." Ninjja wanted to avoid looking at the feeding tube that had been inserted a day ago. She turned away and stepped out of the room to find the doctor on night duty. She allowed them the liberty of a few seconds. The mask was lifted for just a few seconds, allowing them to dab water with a cotton ball on his mouth. The sight of his parched lips was never going to let Ninjja be at peace with herself.

Ninjja's father was trying to say something, but the overzealous attendant shoved the mask back between them as a barrier. The dumb charade continued for the next couple of hours. They were happy that he was fully conscious and was able to express himself. He lovingly hugged both the girls and smiled at their mother. Ninja was so overwhelmed with emotion that she rested her head on his chest the same way as she had as a child, and she found the same comfort when he put his hand over her head. Even in his utterly fragile state, Ninjja felt that his comforting arm around her shielded her from the brutal world outside.

Time was slipping by, and it was time for the attendant to complete his to-do list. He asked the family to step outside, as he wanted to go about sponging the patient. "We will step aside and let you do your job. We won't disturb you at all," the sisters pleaded earnestly to him. He didn't budge at all. They continued to steal more time and tried explaining to their father that they would need to leave for some time. He shook his head vehemently in protest. He gestured with both his hands for them to stay. The attendant was also somewhat moved, but he continued to push. "He will feel better after the cleanup...and it won't take long." He made a convincing pitch.

Ninjja's mother seemed glued to his side. She didn't want to leave him alone. Unfortunately, the attending nurse managed to win over the weary minds of the family. "Don't you worry; I will call you as soon as I am done," he said in a very compassionate and genuine tone.

Ninjja felt that her mind was losing its ability to think and make decisions. The rest of her family was in the same boat. They kissed her father's forehead with a promise to return soon and walked out like zombies.

Outside in the waiting area, Ninjja was stuck in time. Oblivious to the seconds that were ticking away, she was waiting for the signal from the nurse to come back. Ninjja's sister, who was feeling edgy, walked past their room and peeped inside from the small glass window. She could see that her father was raising both his hands as though he was trying to say something. The attending nurse was comfortably sitting on the chair beside him. She had the urge to go inside again to check on him. She reached out for the doorknob... but then held back lest she should upset the nurse. He had given a stern warning earlier not to disturb him while he was doing his job. With reluctance, she pulled herself back and then found a spot next to Ninjja. No words were spoken.

"Ninjja, it has been a long time...I think it has been over an hour and a half." Ninjja's sister finally broke her state of paralysis. The usual routine of chasing, requesting, screaming, and cajoling ensued. An hour later, they were back in their so-called private room. Ninjja was disheartened to see her father in a deep sleep. There was no response to their talking or touching. The hopes of continuing their communication had come to a grinding halt.

• • •

"What were they doing for so long? He was communicating with us when they threw us out...and now they have given him back to us when he is probably unconscious." Ninjja's voice held a lot of pain. Her sister reached out to hold his hand and was shocked to see that it was swollen and covered in bandages.

Her heart sank further when she looked at the blood-pressure monitor. The dramatic change that she witnessed was too overwhelming to handle. She rushed out of the room and burst out into sobs. Ninjja was close at her heels and made a vain attempt at consoling her. With tears streaming from her own eyes, it was difficult to say something that would lessen the grief that her sister was submerged in. After several moments of silence and holding on to each other, they found their bearings. They donned their brave faces again and walked back in to face their mother, who seemed devoid of any emotion. She had turned into stone. The environment around her didn't seem to have any impact.

Soon after, the doctor came on his regular round and pronounced that the end was near. "Doctor! He had improved dramatically at night. He was fully conscious for over two hours till we were thrown out…he was able to move his hands and feet…and then we don't know what happened for the next three hours…and this is how we got him back…" Ninjja expressed her immense grief and frustration.

"In such cases, the situation can change dramatically fairly quickly. Whatever you experienced last night must have been a flicker before the lamp goes out…everything can't be explained." The doctor brushed off her concern.

"I really wish I could have taken him back home late at night…at least we would have been by his side all along," Ninjja continued in a desolate tone.

"With the progress in medical science, all of us are going to die in an ICU!" The doctor made his final comment. Harsh as it sounded, there was some element of hard-hitting truth in it as well.

It was too painful to just watch a dear one gradually sink. The insignificance of human endeavors in the cosmos couldn't be starker than at this moment.

Half an hour later, the physiotherapist came by for his regular procedure of cleaning up the breathing tract. While he was getting ready to insert his contraption, Ninjja's sister spoke out aloud in pain and exasperation, "What is the point of doing all this? Aren't you aware of what the doctor said? Can't we just let him be? And don't poke him anymore! You can put a tick against your visit if you want to…"

Sure enough, the statement did prick the human conscience of the mechanized medical practitioner. His expression gave away a flicker of guilt and sorrow. Immediately he dropped his tools and walked away without another word.

The recent episode took Ninjja's disgust for the system, which unfortunately had the word "care" associated with it, to an entirely new level.

* * *

The dark cover of gloom had sealed Ninjja's ability to think, speak, or act. The other two family members were in the same state. "What if he can hear us?" Ninjja's sister suddenly spoke.

Then Ninjja heard her mother's voice for the first time in the past five hours. "If we sit here quietly, he will think he is all alone."

"Yes, we must talk to him. Let him know that we are here with him…we can probably play his favorite music," Ninjja said.

It was amazing how this simple belief that he was able to hear them kept them going for hours to come. No one from the medical staff had bothered to tell them about the typical condition of the human mind and body at this stage, and it didn't matter to the family any more! The only extraneous things that they had to ward off now were the trainee nurses being sent to administer medicines.

Nine hours later…the inevitable happened. They could do nothing but watch helplessly. They were holding his hands with their full might, but that wasn't enough to keep him back. They could see him slipping from their grip with every passing moment. The monitor and the doctor gave the final decree.

Ninjja was tormented by a tornado of grief, but nothing came out through the eyes. The tears had a dry spell. Fortunately, the family had the support of neighbors and some of Ninjja's friends to help them with the next sets of procedures.

· · ·

After taking hold of her emotions, an hour later, Ninjja was seated at the billing desk to clear her dues. The billing person was sympathetic while producing the reams of pages of invoice.

Ninjja just looked at the final five-figure number and reached out for her credit card. While she was handing over the card, it struck her that the summary sheet did not indicate the senior-citizen discount that the billing desk had voluntarily told her about during admission to ICU. In the moment of grief, it seemed really petty to even think about it.

But maybe that is what they are trying to take advantage of, her subconscious warned her. She had been disgusted enough already with the callousness and the attitude of making money while there was any semblance of life. Extending it further, to make money off a dead man, really took the cake.

Anger and frustration now growled with their fangs in full bloom. She didn't care if people thought of her as a selfish, stingy daughter who couldn't let go of money even in the moment of grief.

Ninjja spoke aloud venomously, just to make a point. "I don't see any senior citizen discount you mentioned…did you think I would not notice?" She fixed her stern gaze on the clerk. The way his facial contours changed clearly gave away that the error had been made on purpose!

His shamed expression gave Ninjja her limited retribution.

· · ·

The day after, Ninjja was overwhelmed to see the number of people who turned up to pay their last respects. "I had no idea that Father had formed so many connections…how did he manage this? For the two years that he has spent in this house, he was mostly unwell and confined to these four walls…such an emotional connection despite so many constraints is unbelievable!" Ninjja couldn't stop herself from making a remark to her mother. There was no response. The sudden vacuum had sealed her lips and dried her tears.

"He was someone who could touch one's heart even in a ten-minute interaction. He was so transparent…so guileless…that there were no barriers that could come in the way…his biggest weakness was also his biggest strength!" Ninjja's sister responded in a faraway tone.

Time was ticking away.

They had to perfunctorily move on to the next steps. Unfortunately, the hospital was not the last one in the chain to make undue profits out of misery.

The ambulance driver suddenly upped his demands after reaching the cremation ground. This was no time for any quibbles. Ninjja was so distraught that her mind didn't even register what was going on. Arv threw the money at the extorting driver with a one-liner— "Hope you know what you are doing"—and rejoined the grieving family without wasting another second.

The Hindu rituals of cremation were heart-wrenching. Before this day, Ninjja had seen some of them only in movies, without understanding how excruciating it could be. It was a sudden catharsis. It looked like they were designed to break the deep bond with a blow. Every step had "let go" written all over it. The act of breaking the earthen pot at the pyre and letting the water flow symbolized the liberation of the spirit. While the connotation was positive, the thud also had the impact of shattering her heart. For a moment, Ninjja could see her own reflection in those broken opaque pieces.

Once back in the car, Ninjja's mother flung her head onto her shoulders and said, "What was he trying to say, when we were thrown out of the room? I keep asking myself. We will never know now…I didn't know then that we would never be able to speak to him again." Her voice was torn. "The feeling that I let him go without hearing him will keep haunting me till the end," she continued with her eyes closed. Ninjja knew that there was an ocean of tears behind those closed eyelids.

"What a moron I have been. I had gone back again to his hospital room and had seen him raise his hands…it looked like he was calling me...I wanted to go in...but I didn't! Why was I so scared of annoying that nurse? What was the downside of getting shunned compared to the priceless gift of giving my father few moments of happiness?" Ninjja's sister brutally admonished herself. Ninjja was equally guilty of not trying again.

"You can't blame yourself. You were just following the instructions after putting forward due resistance. We all thought that it was for the best under the circumstances...and how could we have known that nurse would take so long, and that we would get our father back like this?" Ninjja tried to console her sister overtly in an attempt to find a plausible reason to overcome her own guilt.

Beneath the surface, she was equally tormented by the guilt pangs of not trying hard enough. The sense of closure was missing. Was it even possible?

While the end was inevitable at some point in time, the precipitous, callous drive toward it had left such deep scars on Ninjja that even a lifetime wasn't going to be enough to heal them.

•　•　•

Six months later, Ninjja was going through the motions of getting ready for work when she noticed the broken strap of her office bag. Grumpily, she started unloading the multitude of belongings to a makeshift carry bag, when her crumpled, yellow diary made a reappearance. Ninjja had completely forgotten about its existence, like many other things that she had lost interest in during the past few months.

As she started turning the weatherworn pages, a decade went through right in front of her eyes. The collection of experiences, open questions, and emotions all started speaking to her. They were asking for more.

"Probably there is a final chapter that is yet to be written. That's why I found it after all this time…who knows?" Ninjja muttered to herself as she shoved it back into her bag.

She knew that she wouldn't be able sleep that night till she had emptied her thoughts onto those crumpled, yellow sheets. Confusion continued to reign supreme, and Ninjja didn't know if she was going to get any relief by pouring out her feelings on a piece of paper.

Ninjja had a flashback to another event around the same time.

The grandmother of one of her close friends passed away in a top-rated hospital. She was brought in for a viral fever, which soon became complicated enough to warrant an ICU admission. The horror stories of her treatment made her own experience pale in comparison. The analytical mind-set of her friend's mother uncovered several dark secrets—one of which was that the hospital had done clinical trials of an unrelated drug without seeking permission from the family.

The hospital didn't have an answer when confronted. The gutsy mother persisted with her desire to fight for justice and collected enough evidence to file a PIL (public interest litigation). She also managed to gather several other affected parties to join her petition. The hospital tried several questionable methods to dissuade the brave heart from fighting her case, and eventually they turned their attention to pressing other levers in the system. Needless to say, she never got her due.

Apart from feeling the pain of her friend's family, Ninjja received an uncomfortable assurance that her experience was not unique. "If such is the state of the ICU of another top-rated hospital, shouldn't I just accept what happened?" Ninjja had often asked herself—but it still didn't put her turmoil to rest.

Unfortunately, Ninjja didn't know the question that she was seeking answers to. *What am I going to scribble in my yellow diary? What good it can possibly do?* she wondered hopelessly.

Suddenly, a few dreadful questions stared in her face.

Was it necessary to take her father to the hospital in the first place? Did she purposely ignore all her previous experience to know that there wouldn't be any question that her father would be shoved in the ICU…and that the chances of a successful outcome were remote? Was she too afraid to be considered guilty by her family, just in case her experiment of keeping him at home had failed? Was hospital admission an easier option under the circumstances? Was this action equivalent to shirking responsibility and passing the buck?

Ninjja was nervous. These questions were too difficult to handle. It felt that she was being put on trial. It was an eerie feeling to find one's own self as the defendant, the witness, and the prosecutor. Was she guilty of putting her father through a painful death? This thought was enough to freeze her in her chair.

A loud, incessant ring on her phone thawed her back to her senses. She was delighted to see Arv's name flashing on it. "I am feeling terrible! Now I know the unspoken question that was responsible for my turmoil." She poured out her desperation without wasting another second.

Arv was taken aback. He had called in a cheerful mood to share a funny incident that had just occurred. Ninjja's response forced him to suddenly change gears for a difficult uphill drive.

After Ninjja's narration ended, there was a long pause. This increased her nervousness further. Her situation was that of a person under trial who was unaware of his crime, yet was so tired of back-and-forth arguments that he wanted nothing but a quick verdict.

"It is not just you!" Arv spoke after a long time. "It is not easy to make such calls," he said sympathetically. "I have seen this happen in my own family. One of my relatives decided to admit her husband to the hospital, as it was getting too difficult to take care of him at home. She was a senior citizen herself, and I can understand if it was hard for her to take care of all his needs. Unfortunately, things didn't ease out for her...the situation got complicated during the hospital stay, and he was shifted to the ICU. A few days later, he was put on a ventilator. The daily costs were very high, with no clarity on the outcome. Some of the family members sheepishly suggested that the ventilator support be discontinued and he be taken home instead to rest peacefully. However, there was another group that felt otherwise. The hospital continued with their stance that the possibility of recovery couldn't be ruled out. For want of any clear decision, the poor old woman was ready to spend all her money to continue with the life support.

"Finally, fifteen days and ten lakhs (twenty thousand USD) later, her husband passed away."

Arv paused for a breath.

Ninjja could feel the pain that the old lady must have gone through. She could only mutter some inaudible words, which Arv took as a cue to continue. "Would you say she was wrong in admitting her husband in the first place? Should she have tested her physical limits to keep him at home?

"Was she wrong in keeping the life support, which possibly extended her husband's suffering? Or was she scared that people might consider her to be a selfish wife who tried to save money when her husband was dying? Was she doing it for her own satisfaction? Or was it to avoid the feeling of guilt by using whatever was medically possible? I don't think there is an easy answer there. Imagine the pressure and adversity under which one has to make such a decision! More likely than not, there will be a reason to regret later, irrespective of the decision."

This statement sent Ninjja back in her memory to a decade ago, when her cousin was faced with a critical decision regarding life support for his newborn. He had spent all his money and was borrowing more to keep a little heart beating. His helplessness, his confusion...all came back to life with a new meaning for Ninjja.

"Unless the whole family can unite to make the difficult choices...and there is confidence that there would be no finger-pointing later on...it is hard to say what was right and what was wrong." Arv paused to see if Ninjja had drawn any solace from his monologue.

She was quiet, but the reality of decision making and the complexity of human psychology had started dawning on her.

"Thanks. I am feeling better," Ninjja responded politely. She gradually changed the topic to more pleasant ones to acknowledge and reward Arv's patience, though her own disposition was still far from cheerful.

As always, they bid adieu with a promise to meet soon.

After dinner, Ninjja was back to fiddling with those crumpled, yellow pages that had caused so much commotion in her mind. She picked up the pen and scribbled her first line: "The ICU dilemma."

—m—

A receiver's perspective on health-care challenges

1. Death of the quintessential family doctor
2. Moral corruption spreading its wings in the medical profession
3. Affordability of health-care
4. Quality of attendants and nurses
5. Availability and credibility of information on alternate cures
6. Indiscreet use and abuse of health-care reimbursements and insurance
7. Primitive home-care services
8. **The ICU dilemma**: If a loved one is very sick, one may not have a choice but to rely on the ICU of a hospital. God forbid, if life support is called upon, one doesn't know how to interpret the seesaw of life. The decision to continue or pull the plug is likely to be the most difficult question one can face. Even taking a second opinion is not

feasible. While the patient's family has legal rights to the reports and prescriptions of an ICU patient, it is not always easy to get access to them.

Unfortunately, if the person concerned is elderly, the risks due to hospital-transmitted infections add to the complexity, raising the odds against survival. Considering improving economic standards, more and more people will have access and the means to use the advanced medical facilities. However, betting on dramatic changes in the way hospitals care for ailing senior citizens would at best be speculative. More and more families will be faced with an unspoken difficult choice-a benign death in home care/hospice, or a painful journey through an ICU that shows a faint promise of life!

In hopeless situations, even if a small glimmer of hope is shown, do we expect people to remove life support from their loved ones?

At the same time, one can't deny that miracles also happen in the ICU!

Emotions are not the right ally for difficult decisions. Where is the unattached, neutral expert when people are faced with real life-and-death choices? Can the health-care system gear up to address this most difficult challenge that is staring at us? Do the doctors have the right training and the right incentives to fulfill this role? Is there a need for an independent advisory body whose representatives can guide the family through this most difficult phase and help their decision making?

—∽∽—

On the following day, Ninjja woke up with a sense of purpose. She was not going to run away from the unpreventable element of everyone's life. *Death is an inevitable truth, so why should we shy away from discussing it?*

Over the past few months, whenever Ninjja's mother had tried to have a conversation on dos and don'ts during her own last stages, Ninjja had always changed the topic or fled the scene. Ninjja had interpreted it as a sign of depression or loss of interest in life rather than prudence.

"What a moron I have been…instead of admiring my mother's courage to have such a tough discussion, I have been shutting her off! The next time around, I will try my best to be more mature about it," Ninjja told herself before jotting down one final point on her lessons in the diary.

—∽∽—

My Survival Mantra

1. Don't assume that your regular physician will always know what is right for you.
2. When in doubt, seek a second opinion.

3. Always have health insurance, and carefully select the plan.

4. Don't rush to a specialist based on your perceived issue.

5. Overseas insurance is not a blank check.

6. A balanced lifestyle holds the secret of many a cure.

7. In emergency situations (e.g., an accident), don't run to the closest hospital.

8. If someone dear to you is admitted to the hospital, don't assume that the nurses and attendants are always right.

9. Several diseases may have stress as the underlying cause.

10. Watch out for medicine addiction!

11. Emotional support is a substitute for some medicines.

12. Don't take medicines in blind faith.

13. There is no utopian health-care system.

14. Childhood diet and lifestyle define a large portion of adult health.

15. Explore alternative therapies before going under the knife if you are not in a time-critical situation.

16. Think before you start making all your health issues public.

17. Proactively share and challenge the context, especially for older patients.

18. **Talking about death should not be considered a taboo**: The ICU dilemma is bound to face us! There isn't an eternal right answer, but acknowledging this brutal truth of life is a first step toward coming to terms with the choices one makes

in crucial times. Having candid discussions proactively on this unsavory topic and making one's preferences known could save a lot of excruciating pain for oneself and one's family. The satisfaction of making the right call for a loved one and then living with it for the rest of one's life can't be realized unless the close family responsible for the decision is in agreement.

—∞—

A month later, Ninjja was feeling much more at peace with herself. The demons inside her had been quelled, and she was able to see things in new light.

She felt it was time to finally put her yellow diary in its resting place. She reached into her bag and fortunately found her decade-long friend in the first shot. Ninjja involuntarily found herself flipping through the crumpled pages before putting them away.

The coincidence of eight and eighteen amused her. She had written about eight key health-care challenges, and her list of lessons that were in the patient's realm of influence was eighteen points long!

I should share this with others rather than putting it to rest, she thought before being interrupted by her phone.

"It's me! Just don't say anything, and listen to me!" Arv spoke feverishly. Ninjja almost froze in place.

"I don't think anyone understands me better than you, Ninjja! Whenever I want to share something, be it good or bad, the first person I think of is you. I have no idea what I was chasing so far...the only person that I would like to spend rest of my life is *you*, Ninjja! I was looking for you in everyone I dated! I wanted to tell you this before I lost courage..." He stopped, almost out of breath.

Now it was Ninjja's turn to gasp for breath. She couldn't believe what she was hearing. After a minute of awkward silence that felt like an eternity, Ninjja found her voice: "Arv, you are my rock whenever I am drowning. But...I don't know what that means for us together...I don't know what triggered you to say all this. Please sleep on whatever you just said. We will speak tomorrow..." Her voice trailed off.

Arv was like a spent force that didn't even have the energy to watch the impact of what it had just done. He didn't utter another word. Finally, they bid adieu, and Ninjja defrosted herself with a thud on the bed.

She stared at the ceiling with millions of dots dancing in front of her.

Finally, she rolled over with a pillow to her side. She closed her eyes. She had a smile on her face. It looked like she was waiting for tomorrow.

Patient's Golden Rule

N injja jotted down the headlines of her eighteen points of "Survival Mantra" as a reminder:

1. Don't assume that your regular physician will always know what is right for you.
2. When in doubt, seek a second opinion.
3. Always have health insurance, and carefully select the plan.
4. Don't rush to a specialist based on your perceived issue.
5. Overseas insurance is not a blank check.
6. A balanced lifestyle holds the secret of many a cure.
7. In emergency situations (e.g., an accident), don't run to the closest hospital.
8. If someone dear to you is admitted to the hospital, don't assume that the nurses and attendants are always right.
9. Several diseases may have stress as the underlying cause.
10. Watch out for medicine addiction!

11. Emotional support is a substitute for some medicines.
12. Don't take medicines in blind faith.
13. There is no utopian health-care system.
14. Childhood diet and lifestyle define a large portion of adult health.
15. Explore alternative therapies before going under the knife if you are not in a time-critical situation.
16. Think before you start making all your health issues public.
17. Proactively share and challenge the context, especially for older patients.
18. Talking about death should not be considered a taboo.

Ninjja was looking for ways to create a "minimum survival kit" that one could remember easily.

This is what she finally wrote:

If you are a patient, then have **"ASPIRATION"** as your golden rule:

- ASK questions about your disease—how long does it take for full recovery? Are there any other side effects that you should watch out for? While treating the disease, will there be other symptoms (e.g., nausea, depression, etc.) that you should be mentally prepared for?
- SHARE your history of any other ailments, allergies, and other current health issues—even if the doctor doesn't ask.

- PRECAUTIONS: Ask about any precautions needed regarding food intake, physical activities to avoid, weather conditions that could be particularly problematic, and so on.
- INTERACTIONS: It's important to check for interactions of the current medication with some of your other regular medications, such as psychiatric medicines, BP medicines, and painkillers.
- RATIFICATION of opinion is critical if (1) any invasive procedure is recommended (not just for surgery but for the invasive tests), (2) treatment has to be started for any major ailment (e.g., TB, cancer, etc.), or (3) treatment is not showing any results or symptoms are not moving in the right direction.
- ALTERNATIVES to the suggested course of action. Sometimes there are different ways of treating the same ailment even within allopathic medicine. The doctor may suggest a particular method based on his or her own experience or comfort factor. It is important to explore before following a course of action. At times the alternative branches of medicine (homeopathy, Ayurveda, etc.) may have a better cure, but you need to find a reliable source through word of mouth or through your own efforts.
- TIME: You need to understand several aspects related to time for the treatment: (1) the time it is going to take to heal; (2) the time for a follow-up checkup or change in dosage/course correction; and (3) if there is no permanent cure and the disease just needs to be managed, it is important to understand how the disease might progress over time, what you should watch out for, things that might help, and so on. This helps the patient and the family be much better prepared mentally to deal with situations that lie ahead.
- INSPIRE confidence in yourself and/or the patient (as the case may be). A positive mind-set is as critical as the right medicine for

getting better. If the family is too stressed to think positively, one shouldn't feel shy about seeking external help (either through extended family or through a professional counselor).

- OWN the issue. You are as much responsible for the line of treatment as are the hospitals or the doctors helping you. Often, patients or their families start holding the doctor completely responsible for whatever happens to them. The truth is that you are the best judge of your condition and strength. For example, if you are being suggested hospitalization for recovery, but you feel confident that your condition can be managed at home, please feel free to discuss this with doctors and make your call. Similarly, being vigilant toward the medication being adminstred by attendants and nurses and raising alarm when something doesn't feel right is equally important.

- NUTRITION: The relevance of adequate nutrition for leading a healthy life can never be sufficiently underscored. Childhood nutrition plays a very critical role in adult health. All parents with young children should take note of this. Similarly, during any major illness, the attention required for following the schedule of medicines should not be allowed to take focus away from nutrition.

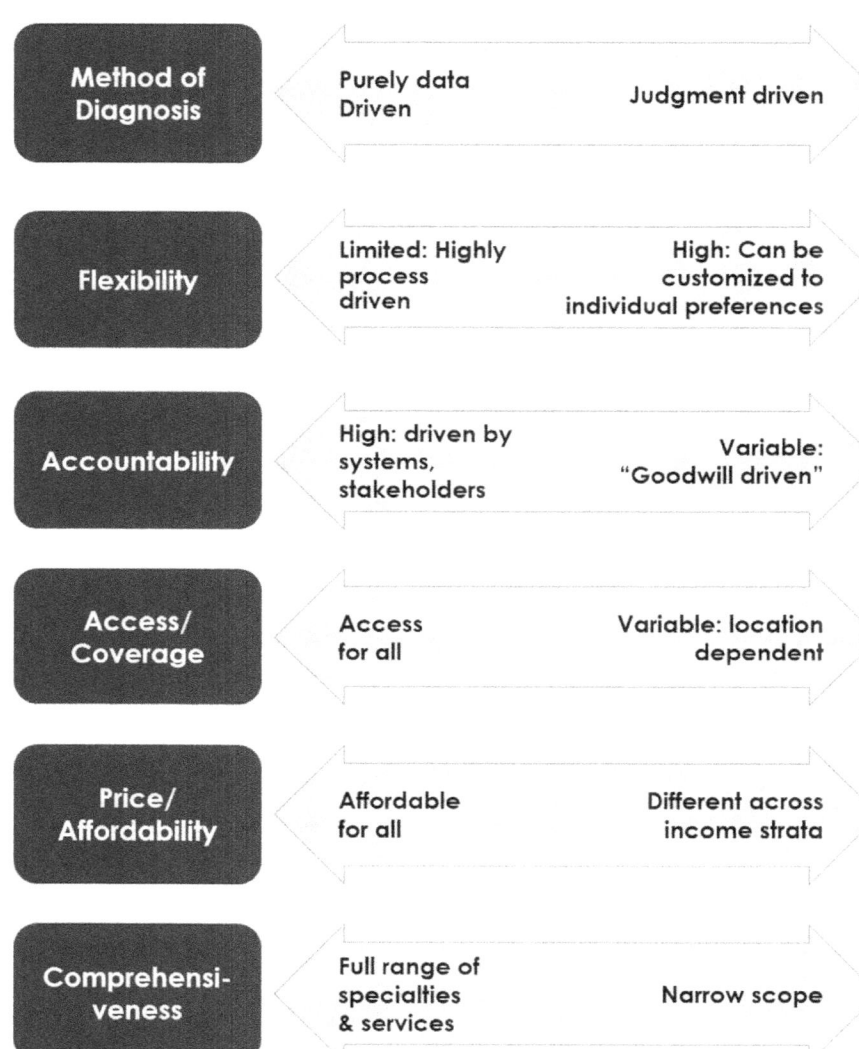

Figure 1: Six key dimensions of trade-offs in different health-care systems

Appendix 1
Constraints, Stakeholders, and Resources for Health-Care Support

Ninjja was clear that the **"Minimum Sufficiency"** should be the goal of providing health-care to the poor. This implied providing the *minimum sufficient* medical intervention such that recovery or disease management through natural courses becomes feasible. Before identifying the solution, it was important to identify the key constraints, stakeholders, and the resources that could be tapped to deliver against this goal.

ADDITIONAL CONSTRAINTS FOR THE LOW-INCOME GROUP

- **Fewer options** to choose from: typically, lower-income individuals would not have the luxury to pay the price of private hospitals (unless there was insurance or they got a cheap loan) and would most likely need to rely on government-funded, charity, or community-funded hospitals.
- **Questionable receptiveness** of the health-care staff to answer questions or course correct (possibly due to strained resources at the health-care provider or due to poor attitude).

- **Financial burden of other related expenses,** such as travel and accommodations to take a patient to the hospital that is best equipped to serve their needs, may be prohibitive.
- **Lack of awareness** about the illness and expectations from the health-care provider—typically, poorer sections of society also have limited exposure to information. Also, their education standards constrain their ability to ask questions and navigate the system.
- **Quality and availability of adequate health-care staff**: given the lower salary levels and difficult working conditions, it may be difficult for the government-funded institutions to attract the right "quality talent" in adequate numbers.
- **Caring for the ill may require an extremely difficult trade-off**: taking one day off from work to take care of a sick family member might be as serious as getting no food for the dependents on that day. Given this context, the illness might be pushed to its full limits before someone consults a doctor. This could compound the moral hazard issue and add more pressure to an already strained system.
- **Cost of medicine could be higher than the cost of consultation**: this could create situations where the patient doesn't follow through a treatment despite having a prescription.
- **Lack of proper methods of financing to the needy**: given that most poor people would not have a track record of their employment, the possibility of getting financing at reasonable rates would be minimal, even if the person had the ability to repay the loan. The chances of such people falling prey to unscrupulous lenders would further exacerbate their situation.
- **The root cause of illness may be beyond the purview of the health-care provider**. The root causes of several illnesses may lie in malnutrition, lack of sanitation standards,

inadequate access to clean drinking water, or overexposure to polluted air (e.g., the urban poor). Even if the illness is cured, the chances of recurrence cannot be ruled out.

RESOURCES IN THE SYSTEM

- Finances from the government
- NGOs, charities, and global agencies focused on health-care
- Sharing or spreading risks across a broader population through medical insurance
- Funds available for family welfare, sanitation, and health

THREE CATEGORIES OF KEY STAKEHOLDERS

- **Good Samaritans**: They target good health outcomes but don't have financial ROI (return on investment) expectations. For example:
    - Government
    - Global welfare agencies like WHO, World Bank, etc.
    - Charities
    - NGOs
    - Some educational/research institutes
- **End users and affected parties**: These are the beneficiaries or the sufferers as the case may be:
    - Less privileged patients and their families
    - Companies or employers of the "poor strata" of society
- **For-profit market participants**: These are market partici-pants that are critical for delivery and make a living out of their participation in this market (hence the financial incentive):
    - Insurance companies
    - Doctors and other health-care professionals

- Medical equipment and technology suppliers
- Some research institutes
- Pharmaceutical companies
- Private hospitals

Appendix 2

Suggested Actions for Key Stakeholders of the Health-Care System

1. STAKEHOLDER 1: "THE GOOD SAMARITANS"

Fortunately, the goal of all the stakeholders in this category seems aligned to getting good health outcomes without worrying about financial returns. They can create the right enabling conditions:

- **Promote healthy collaboration** between private partici-pants and the donors through a framework of public-private partnership, not just for building hospitals and clinics, but also for creating conditions to avoid the spread of diseases in the first place (e.g., access to clean water, sanitation, hygiene, preventive checks, etc.).

    Evidence suggests that it is possible to develop viable and effective models for such a collaboration. With $3.8 tril-lion in government spending (of the total $6.5 trillion globally on health-care), these stakeholders indeed seem well posi-tioned to define the direction of the funds' flow, dictate tar-get outcomes, and influence the efficacy of deployment. To not use their privileged position to set the direction should at best be called a "stupor" if not a "coma."

- **Add results/outcome metrics** instead of stipulating input parameters. Typically, the funding agencies and governments provide guidelines, like percentage of expense to be funded by government, salary of staff, cost of treatment for each disease, and so on, which sometimes distort incentives and create a suboptimal result for the system.

  Instead, outcome metrics for the system as well as at the individual level are likely to direct efforts more appropriately. Some of the system-level metrics could be tracking healthy life years, incidence of hygiene related diseases, self-perceived level of health, distribution of population health outcomes, and so on. Even for the metrics at the individual unit level (e.g., hospitals), a lot of literature exists, but the actual reporting is, at best, patchy.

  Some easier metrics, like death rate for certain diseases, are tracked more regularly, but they don't do justice to measuring the effectiveness and efficiency of treatment. Lead indicators like percentage of pneumonia cases that got treated without hospital admission, cost of tests before accurate diagnosis is made, thirty-day readmission rate, and so on could be more valuable in optimizing scarce resources.

  While statisticians could argue about standardization or the best methodology of measurement, this is not reason enough to not make a beginning somewhere.

- **Prioritize prevention.** Prevention of diseases should find a topmost slot in the policy framework. It is estimated that over 2.5 million deaths of children under five could be prevented through proper sanitation and clean water. Additionally, almost half of ailments among the poor in developing economies could be linked to malnutrition, lack of access to clean water, poor sanitation, and inadequate hygiene standards. This is enough evidence to suggest that investments in prevention are likely to offer much more rewarding returns.

Significant efforts for preventive medicines for developing countries (including support for innovation, research, and development) to find cost-effective solutions are already underway by organizations like the WHO, but will these be sufficient? Changes in the mind-set of health-care providers will be equally important. For example, if a doctor chooses to ignore (or doesn't have the skills to understand) some early symptoms of a deadly disease, all the efforts spent in creating a preventive cure will come to naught. Some portion of funds should also be directed toward actions (e.g., random audits or training) that embed good behavioral disciplines.

- **Link funding with performance and create transparency.** At the risk of stating the obvious, it would be extremely important to tie the level of funding to demonstrated performance of the partners. While the record of performance-linked support to pharmaceutical companies is more notable, the same can't be said of the clinics and hospitals that have a critical role as the "last mile" in health-care delivery. The pilots have certainly shown promise, but it would take a joint commitment of the Good Samaritans to move the needle on the ground. Additionally, a portion of funding should be directed toward promoting e-platforms. This should enable transparency in tracking the deployment of funds and tying it to the physical inventory, as well as help in plugging the giant hole that is created by leakages in the system.

- **Create awareness** among people about inputs for healthy living:

  Unfortunately, a large portion of the 2.5 billion people in the world who don't have access to sanitation are not even aware that they are living at the pithead of diseases.

While creating access to improved water, sanitation, and hygiene standards might logically be part of government departments other than health, the common goal of well-being should unite them. The Good Samaritans can play an important role in creating the right linkage and aligning the efforts and direction of funds to create more awareness.

- **Regulatory support to ensure every citizen is health-care enabled.** There are enough thought papers on the issue of providing health insurance coverage to the poor or on creating a health-care corpus and the like.

  Several interesting ideas, like managed-care health-insurance plans, risk pooling, and community-based insurance, have shown some success, at least at a small scale, proving that it is possible to have a for-profit model even while serving the poor.

  Why don't we see them in practice? One can attribute this phenomenon to the boon and the bane of an emerging market. In the early days, there is enough opportunity to cream the top layer and make much higher profits without having to worry about a deeper reach. It is natural for the other segments (less profitable ones) to get deprioritized in early days. Given the uncertainties involved and the limitation on resources, any sensible business manager would focus on the top end for maximizing profits.

Free enterprise cannot always be the panacea. Happy marriage of social requirements with business motives isn't possible without the right regulatory framework.

If the mere mention of "national security" wakes up even the somnambulists in the policy makers, then how about securing the health of our people? Does it occupy the same high spot in our thinking? Isn't high time we really raised the game on this?

2. STAKEHOLDER 2: END USERS AND AFFECTED PARTIES

The end users (patients) and affected parties (family, employers) of the financially weaker strata can't be just silent observers. Thinking that they are just the recipients without any control over their destiny would be nothing short of a defeatist mentality. Several actions are under their control:

- **Take advantage of preventive health-check camps** offered by NGOs and publicly funded hospitals. More often than not, the poor are not even aware of the value of preventive checks. The reach of television and mobile phones should be exploited for spreading the word.
- **Watch out for sanitization** standards, personal hygiene, and cleanliness of surroundings. While it is very easy to blame the government or local authorities for a poor state of cleanliness, the community's vital role cannot be ignored. If people choose to dump garbage at their doorstep every waking moment, it is preposterous to assume that the government could keep it clean.

  Consider the case of the transformation of the industrial city of Surat in India after an outbreak of a lethal disease in 1994. A case study, *Transformation of Surat from Plague to Second Cleanest City in India by H. M. Shivanand Swamy, et al"* summarises it well. Surat at that time could easily compete for the title of filthiest city in the country. It was jokingly referred to as the city "floating on garbage," given the clogged drainages and inadequate access to solid-waste disposal. The outbreak of the disease (which resembled plague), created a panic. Hundreds died, and thousands suffered prolonged hospital stays to save their lives. Needless to say, this small industrial and trading town suffered huge emotional and financial losses (the loss just due to people fleeing the city was estimated at $300 million). The new municipal commissioner took on the challenge and created a model of inclusive urban governance.

Spurred on by his initiative, citizens realized the burning need to clean up the city and came forward to offer full support (which at times meant letting go of unauthorized construction to make way for road-widening or draining systems). The NGOs and local volunteers augmented the public machinery willingly. Within a couple of years, the city attained the position of the second-cleanest city in the country. The city also ranked fourth in a global study of fastest-developing cities conducted by the City Mayors Foundation, an international think tank on urban affairs. Even after close to two decades, the city has maintained its spot as the third-cleanest city in India—a distinction that cannot be sustained without sustained action from the citizens."

Even in the rural areas and in the slums in the backyards of megacities, one can see some bright spots, depending on the awareness and the initiative that the community takes.

- **Create a personal health-care fund:** In most cultures, there is always something that is considered sacred or is critical enough to save for. As an example, it is well understood that even the poorest of the poor start saving for the wedding of their girl child in India. Some of the more progressive ones start saving for the education of their male child. Some others save for a pilgrimage. The question really is, where does health fit in our hierarchy? One needs to learn to treat health at par (if not more) than the corpus that they keep aside for some of these sacred and critical priorities.
- **Employers can play an important role in making the informal sector employees "health-care enabled."** Going back to the case of the housemaid discussed earlier—where

the estimated financial loss due to lower productive life could be $10,000 to $20,000—wouldn't she be willing to make a contribution toward securing her future if she were aware of this equation? Would it be so hard to convince the same maid in question, who was happy spending five to ten dollars per month on her mobile phone, to budget for her own well-being? The employers could top up the maid's contribution to create a further incentive. Ninjja remembered her old maid, Taira, who had found a small corner in the shoe rack of her apartment as a storage space to save money for a rainy day. It had been a chance discovery for Ninjja.

She was moved to see that her maid thought that the money would be safer in Ninjja's house than in her own shanty. With availability of zero-balance accounts for the lower-income groups, along with online money transfer facilities, it should be possible to safely create a corpus. This could be used up for preventive care, for buying health insurance, or for any other health emergency. This is just one idea. There could be a million other possibilities that could work more effectively in different contexts.

- **Create awareness in one's own sphere of influence.** One could argue that the underprivileged might not be able to appreciate the idea that they also have an important role to play in their own health, as most of them are uneducated and blissfully unaware. The concern is genuine, but we need to push the boundaries. How about a viral approach for spreading the word?

STAKEHOLDER 3: FOR-PROFIT MARKET PARTICIPANTS

To understand the preferences of the "for-profit" participants, along the two dimensions of "Type of Health-Care Support" versus

"Customer's Ability to Pay", Ninjja made a pictorial representation, as shown below:

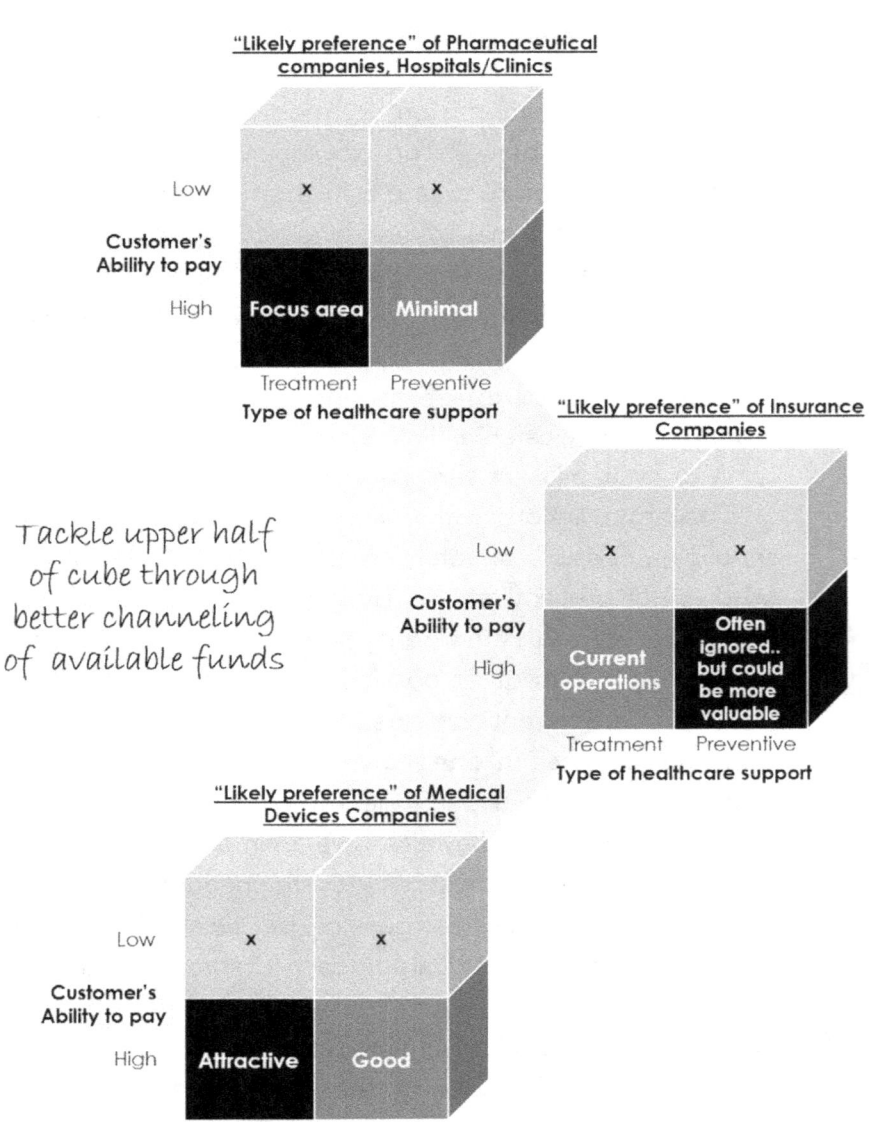

Clearly, there were segments that were not in the consideration set, but given the support from "Good Samaritans" to improve health status for society and the need to ensure longer-term sustainability of their own businesses, several win-win initiatives were possible:

- **Proactive approach to PPP (public-private partnership)**: Proactively shape the public-private partnership options to fill the gap in the ability to pay. Private players could bring much-needed efficiency to health-care delivery, and governments could benefit from more rapid expansion than would not be feasible otherwise. Support in the form of cheaper land, regulatory approvals, and partial funding of treatment given to the less privileged could help develop viable models if the private players keep to the boundary conditions defined for them. This could be a win-win situation: private-market players get to expand the market for themselves and make money, and the governments and funding agencies get the efficiency, speed, and reach in serving the poor.

- **Attack the cost curve**: Follow the minimum-sufficiency principle to service a large segment that has been left out of the pool for most practical purposes. This would also improve the well-being of the privileged class by saving them from the problem of overmedication.

  Attacking the cost curve doesn't necessarily mean losing out on profit. In several other industries, new challengers have come in and changed the rules of the game.

  Ninjja remembered the purchase of her first mobile phone. She had shelled out two months of her salary to buy a heavy, clumsy mobile phone out of sheer necessity back then. To top it all, the usage charge was an exorbitant forty cents per minute, making the phone such a precious commodity that it was fit only to serve the purpose of wartime radio messaging. After a decade and a half, the mobile phone was now affordable to even a daily laborer; the cost of purchase had decreased to one-twentieth, and the usage cost had decreased to one-fiftieth. And interestingly, all the operators were making a lot more money. They were benefiting from economies of scale as well as additional services (like data). Ninjja started thinking about a few other industries and realized that computers, cameras, TVs, and cars had all evolved from eclectic to mass market.

If we are not seeing such dramatic changes in health-care, it may not be because of design but rather because of choice. The good news is that necessity can force the choice to change.

- **Create new, innovative products**: If the focus of efforts of pharma companies (R&D, new product launch, sales and distribution, etc.) could be reoriented toward prevention, suddenly the world of health-care would start looking very different.

  Similarly, different health-insurance products that actually encourage preventive checks, reimburse a percentage of consultation charges, and promote awareness to improve health would need to be created. It could stop the need for crisis intervention at the hospital and potentially turn a loss-making venture profitable for several insurance companies, as well as for government-run hospitals.

  Medical-device companies would need to focus on creating no-frills options for the masses. *Are the funds available to kick-start the process?* She looked at the data again.

Spending on health-care averages at about 10 percent of GDP globally. The wealthy United States spent over 17 percent of its GDP, with poorer Asia and Africa spending around 4–6 percent. The total expenditure on health (including private expenses) globally is a sizeable US $6.5 trillion. The much-vilified pharmaceutical companies and medical-devices industry account for relatively small share with their combined size of US $1 trillion. This implies that bulk of the expenditure goes into services (hospitals, clinics, etc.) and into the much-talked-about leakages and waste.

Even if only 10 percent of leakage and waste could be plugged through the involvement of the private sector, better controls, and so on, suddenly funds upward of US $650 billion would become available through this lever alone to support the subsidy, changes, and innovations required.

Indeed, there would be some redistribution of wealth. It would cannibalize some portion of the highly lucrative treatment segment due to fewer inpatient stays, fewer complicated procedures, and fewer emergencies. But the business of preventive care—diagnostics, nutrition, lifestyle management, and so on—could grow dramatically. New business segments would open up while improving the health quotient.

Ninjja's strong belief that anything that was in the best interest of society created economic value was affirmed.

Shortsightedness and selfish motives would not go away in this new world that Ninjja was visualizing. She hoped that a healthy tension created by competitive forces, regulations, funding agencies, and pressure from customers would force the system to work in a desired fashion.

Bibliography

Bloom, D.E., D. Canning, and J. Sevilla. 2004. "The Effect of Health on Economic Growth: A Production Function Approach." World Development 32(1): 1–13.

Borlaug, Norman E. "The Green Revolution Revisited and the Road Ahead." Lecture, Norwegian Nobel Institute, Oslo, September 2000.

Center on the Developing Child at Harvard University "The Foundations of Lifelong Health Are Built in Early Childhood." *http://www.developingchild.harvard.edu,* 2010.

Clements, Benedict, David Coady, and Sanjeev Gupta. *The Economics of Public Health Care Reform in Advanced and Emerging Economies.* Washington, DC: IMF, 2012.

Dimovska, Donika, Stephanie Sealy, Sofi Bergkvist, and Hanna Pernefeldt. *Innovative Pro-Poor Healthcare Financing and Delivery Models.* Washington, DC: Results for Development Institute, 2009

Wingfield, Claire, Christenson Kaitlin, *Financing and Coordination of Health Research. Perspectives from Nonprofits on Accelerating Product Development and Improving Access for Low- and Middle-Income Countries.* Vol. 2. Washington, DC: Global Health Technologies Coalition, 2013.

Glassman, Amanda, and William Savedoff. "The Health Systems Funding Platform: Resolving Tensions between the Aid and

Development Effectiveness Agendas." Working Paper 258. Washington, DC: Center for Global Development, 2011

Goguen, Frank J., and John D. Connolly. *Global Wealth Creation: The Impacts on Emerging Markets' Health Care*. BostonThe Boston Company Asset Management, LLC, 2012

Kaplan, Warren, Veronica J. Wirtz, Aukje Mantel-Teeuwisse, Pietr Stolk, Beatrice Duthey, and Richard Laing. *Priority Medicines for Europe and World—July 2013 Update*. Geneva, Switzerland: WHO Press, 2013

Kelley, Robert *Where Can $700 Billion in Waste Be Cut Annually from the US Healthcare System?* : Thomson Reuters, 2009.

Kilpatrick, C., B. Allegranzil, and D. Pittet. *WHO First Global Patient Safety Challenge: Clean Care Is Safer Care, Contributing to the Training Of Health-Care Workers around the Globe*, WHO: Geneva, Switzerland, 2011.

Lewis, Maureen. "Governance and Corruption in Public Health Care Systems." Center for Global Development, Working Paper Number 78, 2006.

"Press Note on Poverty Estimates Government of India." Planning Commission, January 2011.

Shivanand Swamy, H. M., Anjana Vyas, and Shipra Narang. *Transformation of Surat from Plague to Second Cleanest City in India*. New Delhi: All India Institute of Local Self Government, 1999.

Stevens, Philip. "Diseases of Poverty and the 10/90 Gap." International Policy Network, London, UK, 2004.

Sudharshan Canagarajah, XiaoYe. "Efficiency of Public Expenditure Distribution and Beyond." Africa Region Working Paper Series, Number 31, 2002.

WHO, *"The World Health Report, Health Systems Financing: The Path to Universal Coverage"*. Switzerland: WHO, 2010.

WHO, *"World Health Report, Working Together for Health."* Switzerland: WHO, 2006.

Supplemental Information

1. The rupee-to-dollar rate has fluctuated during the decade described in this book. For the sake of simplicity, a conversion rate of 50 to 1 USD has been used.
2. The numbers in the book are indicative. The specifics will vary depending on the source and the exact period. However, they can be used to get a sense of the order of magnitude or relative proportions.
3. Refer to the discussion on penetration of health insurance in chapter 2. The statistics quoted are during the time period of when this conversation takes place. Since then the penetration of health insurance has changed:
   a. Over a decade, it has increased marginally in India: Different sources put the latest estimate at approximately 15 percent.
   b. The most remarkable progress has been observed in China, which has gone from under 25 percent penetration in 2004 to over 90 percent in 2010.
4. With respect to the discussion on leakages in health-care funds, it is difficult to assign an accurate number. However, various proxies and pilot studies indicate that this is a serious enough challenge, especially for developing economies.

Example: Canagarajah Ye traces the different points of resource distribution in Ghana and measures the leakage. As per the Transparency International website, World Bank surveys show that in some countries, up to 80 percent of nonsalary health funds never reach local facilities. A WHO fact sheet (Fact sheet N°335 December 2009), "Medicines: corruption and pharmaceuticals" indicates that in some developing countries up to 89% leakage of procurement and operational costs has been observed. In some other reports and news coverage, similar higher numbers are quoted.

5. Regarding the discussion on viral methods of spreading the message (in chapter 6), the definition of middle class is considered to be a family with an annual income between 3.4 lakhs to 17 lakhs (at 2009–10 price levels) as per the National Council for Applied Economic Research's (NCAER) Centre for Macro Consumer Research. A conservative estimate of 35 million households was considered based on the information on actuals at the time of writing this book: 31.4 million middle-class households and 3.2 million higher-income households. This number is estimated to be more than 50 million by 2015–16.

6. The discussion in Appendixes 1 and 2 on constraints and potential actions draws on various papers published on this subject by agencies like WHO, IMF, USAID, CDC, and the author's own perspective.

7. Appendix 2 offers a discussion on sanitation—UNICEF and WHO jointly set the water, sanitation and hygiene goals, targets, and indicators and publish periodic reports. As their report suggests, there have been significant improvements; however, there is still much to be done.

8. Public-information sources that were extensively consulted are listed below:

www.who.int (World Health Organization)

http://www.cdc.gov/ (Centers for Disease Control and Prevention)

http://www.oecd.org/ (The Organisation for Economic Cooperation and Development)

http://kff.org (The Henry J. Kaiser Family Foundation)

http://www.ncaer.org/ (The National Council for Applied Economic Research's (NCAER) Centre for Macro Consumer Research)

http://www.mohfw.nic.in/ (Ministry of Health and Family Welfare, Govt. of India)

https://www.irda.gov.in/ADMINCMS/cms/Uploadedfiles/ IRDA_Handbook_2010-11_Full_Report.pdf (Handbook on Insurance Statistics, 2010–11, Insurance Regulatory and Development Authority of India)

Author Bio

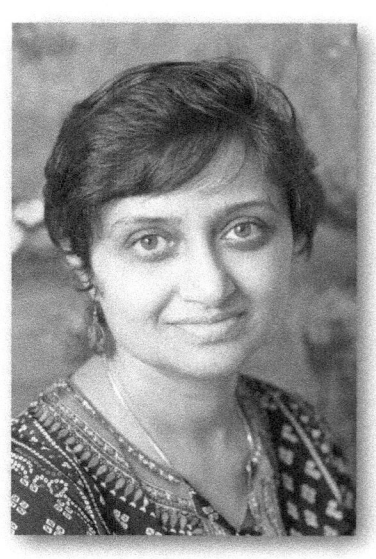

Neelam Phadke is an engineer from Indian Institute of Technology, New Delhi and MBA from Kenan-Flagler, University of North Carolina. She has more than two decades of experience with two of the top three global strategy consulting firms and leading corporates. A world traveler, she has lived in both the United States and India, where she currently resides, and has firsthand experience of both countries' health-care systems. A strong believer in holistic approach to health, she often relies on life-style changes and herbs from her own organic farm as a complement to medical advice to overcome health-hiccups. Trained to consider problems objectively, she chose to use her bittersweet experiences to highlight the challenges of dealing with the health-care web and share her survival tips by compiling her findings into *The Ninjja Sutra*.

www.ingramcontent.com/pod-product-compliance
Lightning Source LLC
Chambersburg PA
CBHW070626290526
45790CB00001B/5

*   9 7 8 1 5 1 1 4 4 6 9 2 1   *